LIFE ROLLS ON

Rich Ochoa
Duane Hale

Published in the United States of America by Rich Ochoa and Duane Hale. Available on amazon.com, bn.com and in Apple iBookstore

ISBN 9781463777586

Second Edition

To Our Families
&
To Billy Brewster (June 9, 1959 – February 18, 1977)
&
To David Wilkerson (May 19, 1931 – April 27, 2011)

Table of Contents

Acknowledgements

We were both thrilled when the cover artwork came back. Viki Bunch created a front and back cover that makes a great first impression on our readers. Her company, *Lasting Impressions by Viki,* based in Duane's hometown of Lindale, TX, does extraordinary photos and artwork and we are lucky that Duane's best friend, Ronald, married someone so talented.

We are indebted to our volunteer editors. Frank Chapchuk, Lindsay Ochoa, Sandra Hale White, Rena Neely, Carrie Fitzgerald, Kyle Vandivort, Wendy Tofani, and the writers at Trinity Writer's Workshop in Bedford, Texas, your critique, editing, and suggestions made this book possible. Top billing goes to our senior editor, Jeff Raimer, who works for nothing more than Hooter's wings.

Thanks to those who helped us develop content and recall facts. Peggy Hale, Kim Hale, Logan Hale, Ronald Bunch, Jimmie Brewster, Sandra White, Lieutenant David Craft, Karen Dickerson, Rene Kennedy, your contributions to the manuscript are immeasurable.

Thanks to our families who understood how important this project was to us and endured three months of our obsession to complete it.

We both wish to acknowledge our hometown of Lindale, Texas. Rich is thankful for that community's support for his first book, *One Way Ticket to Anywhere*. Duane cannot begin to express his gratitude to the people in town who have been there for him his whole life.

Author's Note

This book is a memoir of Duane's life thus far. It represents a tiny sliver of the full story that began over forty-six years ago. Our task was to condense it and present it in a way that will take the reader a few hours to read. Although it is a work of nonfiction, some names have been changed and some characters are composites. We make no claim that the dialog attributed to characters represents a word-for-word record of events. No one could possibly recall unrecorded dialog verbatim. Nonetheless, we constructed the narrative and scenes striving for authenticity in the facts, moods, and feelings of the moments.

Writing a book like this presents unique technical challenges to its coauthors. The point-of-view must be clear and not confuse the reader. This is the story of a man who has achieved so much that we would consider "normal" despite a severe handicap that worsens with years. So inspiring are these accomplishments that a first-person account of them might sound self-aggrandizing. Therefore, most of the book is written in third person in the voice of coauthor, Rich Ochoa.

There are some chapters and sections that call for a first-person narrative. We want the reader to be in

Duane's mind—to BE Duane—and we think the best way to do this is to feature Duane's voice without an intermediary. Those passages are presented with Duane's name as an *italicized* chapter sub-title or section header.

Regardless of whose voice or point-of-view a particular chapter is written in, both writers contributed to every sentence. Duane can still write. He once used a keyboard; now he lays back and moves a mouse across his stomach to click characters one-by-one on a display-based keyboard as he writes his journal.

Rich took Duane's journal entries and his own notes based on hundreds of hours of telephone conversations and bedside discussions and created the chapters and stories. Duane proofread them, added missing details and noted any inaccuracies or embellishments that needed editing. It was an iterative process that went back and forth many times during the development of every chapter.

Another challenge in presenting this story was laying out the sequence of the chapters. The book is mostly chronological, but to maintain topic flow we employed some time jumping. In doing so, we tried to differentiate between the past and present. It's important for the reader to understand that some scenes or chapters set years ago depict Duane engaging in activities he cannot perform today. Although this book may put him in a wheelchair on page forty and have him walking on page sixty, the most hideous aspect of Duane's disease is that his body never gets better, it only gets worse.

We also want readers to know that twenty percent of net royalties from the sale of this book will be dedicated to Logan's college fund. Just in case Logan's baseball skills don't pave his way through college, this book is part of our backup plan to send him to school. If you enjoy it tell your friends.

One other thing: We used thirteen-point font, instead of twelve. It was Duane's idea. On top of everything else, his eyes have always been bad, and he wants as many people as possible to be able to read the book.

Introduction

"I used to come home every night and complain that my feet hurt. After reading this book, I'm gonna quit complaining."
--Gene Williams (rep for publisher of Life Rolls On)

Think back to when you woke up this morning. Imagine how different your day would be if you couldn't move your body. You wanted to scratch the overnight crust from your eyes, but you couldn't. You weren't able to use the restroom or splash water on your face. You couldn't even turn an inch in your bed to get more comfortable. Wonder for a moment how different your life and your family's life would be if you lived every moment of every day without muscles. Wonder what it would be like to be Duane Hale.

Duane has Spinal Muscular Atrophy, SMA. About one in ten thousand babies are born with the condition. It's the number one genetic killer of children under two years old. Because the symptoms and effects endured by the victim are similar, SMA is often considered a member of a better-known family of diseases, Muscular Dystrophy.

From the day he was born, SMA prevented Duane's body from producing motor neuron proteins in his spinal cord. The absence of developed motor neurons means commands from his brain don't make it all the way to his muscles. As a result, the fibers within his muscles slowly wither away from lack of use.

In the physical sense, Duane at forty-six can do only a small fraction of the things he used to do. If you made a list of a hundred random action verbs you'd probably find that at some point in his life, Duane has done about eighty of them. When he celebrated his forty-sixth birthday he might have been able to do about ten of those eighty without assistance.

Those who are acquainted with him but not extremely close (a category I fell into when I began this project) might find his story enlightening because of the perception we have when we see Duane in public. If you see him all dressed up, smiling, buzzing around in his wheelchair, you might get the impression that he can do just about anything we can do except stand up and walk. If you extend your hand to invite Duane to shake, you'll find out that he can't reciprocate your gesture. Instead he makes a fist and offers a fist bump.

To casual observers who see him in that way over the course of many years it may seem like nothing changes. Make no mistake; Duane's condition has worsened with time. In junior high, he could raise a trumpet to his lips and hold it there for five minutes and play. Today he can't even raise his hand to his mouth while sitting in his wheelchair. Even as you read this book his body continues to deteriorate as he loses even more functionality.

He can see, hear, smell, breathe, chew, blink, swallow, and move his right arm through a very limited range that allows him to perform a few other basic tasks. Oh…and anyone who knows him knows that he can talk—nonstop. Other than that he can't do much else with his body.

For now, his fingers are strong enough to push a joystick on his wheelchair. Someday, if he lives long enough, he won't even be able to do that.

Duane lives in the present—a confluence of the past and the future. He has spent his whole life with the knowledge that his condition is worse in that present than it's ever been in the past, yet better than it will ever be in the future.

How does someone live like that and find happiness in spite of such enormous challenges? How does one not only keep from going mad but smile, laugh, and joke along the way?

Even as the disease paralyzes more of his body every day his spirit stays strong and Life Rolls On.

Duane Walks Funny

It was October, 2002, and I was back in Lindale, Texas for the first time in many years to attend my twenty-year class reunion. I found myself driving through a town I barely recognized. Some of the same buildings were still there but they served different purposes. The seven units of the one-time Bonny Motel were now home to small businesses such as a computer repair shop and an insurance company. Tindel's Drug Store had become a knickknack shop.

I got out of my car and walked around town. The faces were unfamiliar but nonetheless, I studied each one briefly as we passed each other on the sidewalk and in the shops, searching for traces of recognition. They looked through me. The people in my hometown were strangers.

I drove up Eagle Spirit Drive to my old high school, but it wasn't a high school anymore. It was some kind of intermediate or elementary school now. I felt disconnected from my hometown. After learning that little kids had taken over my old high school, I planned to head back out of town toward the reunion event when my eyes caught a familiar form on the other side of Highway 69. Across the street was an electric wheelchair moving away from me down a residential road. I saw the back of the full, round head of its driver jutting above the back support of the chair. I made a left turn and watched the man in the chair from a different angle before he disappeared behind Lindale Lumber Company. The erect posture and stoic profile looked familiar. *I wonder if that's—*

No, that's ridiculous. Duane wouldn't be around anymore.

Even though logic told me it was unlikely that I knew the man in the wheelchair, I looped back around to get a closer look. I drove up slowly, approaching him from behind, following in the path of the chair for a bit until I pulled up beside him. He turned his head to look at me. I couldn't believe what I was seeing. The man in the wheelchair was a grownup version of a kid I knew in high school—more than an acquaintance, not quite a friend. Until that very moment I had assumed Duane Hale had long since passed away from Muscular Dystrophy.

We each pulled over to the side of the road. I got out of my car and walked toward him. A boyish, big smile spread across the face of the man who nearly twenty-five years ago liked to take pictures of me pole vaulting. He greeted me by emphatically announcing my name. "Rich Ochoa!"

I felt as though I was standing before a ghost. "Duane! I thought you were… I mean, I thought that was you!" Instinctively, I reached down to shake his hand.

He pivoted his forearm at the elbow, which rested on the armrest of his wheelchair, raising his hand just a little, presenting it in response to my handshake invitation more like a woman in the movies who wants it kissed in the ritual of a formal introduction. I held his flabby hand in mine and wiggled it up and down awkwardly. We made small talk for a minute or two before he suggested that we move the conversation from the side of the road to his living room, which was just fifty yards ahead.

The man who hadn't walked in twenty-five years, who couldn't lift two pounds, put me at ease instantly with humor. "My house is a little messy. If I had known you were coming I would've vacuumed and scrubbed the floors."

My old classmate talked about his job as a police dispatcher and his wife, Kim, but most of all he rambled on with pride about his young son, Logan. He showed me pictures of a boy who looked just like him. *How can this be?* "You have a son?"

Duane sensed my ignorance and shock. He must have been accustomed to explaining to people. "Oh yeah. All that works," he said with a mischievous smile, a nod and wink. "You probably noticed the disease has made me weaker, but I'm still kicking."

Actually, I hadn't noticed. Maybe it's because I hadn't paid close attention back then. *He was in a wheelchair then. He's in a wheelchair now. What difference would I notice?*

As I sat in Duane's house catching up with him about our lives and what became of the kids we knew, I strained for specific childhood memories of him. I recalled something I thought he would find funny. "Duane, I remember when I first saw you. You were in seventh grade—" I paused and collected my thoughts. I looked at this man who had achieved so much despite the challenges God put before him, a man who sat in his wheelchair smiling so big, obviously so happy and proud to have me in his home. I was too ashamed to finish telling the story. Even though I didn't tell Duane, the sudden memory of the event that I had repressed for twenty-five years didn't make it any less real. It took me nine years and an agreement to write this book together to finally tell him this story.

I saw Duane Hale for the first time when his seventh grade class entered Lindale Junior High. On the first day of school, I was part of a group of eighth graders who were chasing down seventh grade boys one-by-one to initiate them into "our school."

We hunted like a wolfpack. We'd separate one of them from the herd, surround the prey and then go in for the kill which consisted of at least one of three welcome-to-junior-high greetings: an atomic wedgie, holding the boy down while we poured a can of soda on his face, or carrying him to the nearest fifty-five gallon drum our school used as trashcans and dropping him into it.

After our mob threw Victor Tennyson, the toughest kid in seventh grade, into a trash can, almost all the seventh grade boys disappeared from the playground. The last boy left was a short kid with blonde, curly hair, big glasses, a scrawny, little body and a round head. Our self-appointed leader, Ronnie Blaylock hollered and pointed toward our next target. "Seventh grader!"

"Yeah, seventh grader!" another agreed. The pack was ready to go. Compared to Victor Tennyson, this kid was gonna be easy.

Then a voice of dissent was heard within our ranks—a voice of reason. Jimmy Kemp spoke up. "No! Wait! Not him."

"Why not him? He's a seventh-grader," Ronnie replied.

Jimmy explained. "That kid is crippled. He can't run or nothin'."

"So, he's still a seventh-grader, ain't he?" Ronnie asked.

A third boy weighed in. "Man, I ain't givin' a wedgie to no crippled kid."

If not for a single voice of compassion in our mini mob, I might have been one of twelve boys who had carried a defenseless kid with Spinal Muscular Atrophy and thrown him into a trashcan that he wasn't capable of escaping.

During those first few weeks of school I noticed the same kid watching us play football on the playground. He paced back and forth alongside our playing field following the game action, but his walk looked goofy. He placed his hands on the small of his back and appeared to push his pelvis forward as he swung his legs seemingly from the hips. He had no knee lift. He looked like he was mocking some old west gunfighter walking in heavy, stiff chaps with his hands on holstered pistols.

I didn't understand that I was watching a twelve-year-old boy valiantly fighting a horrific disease. I thought he was clowning around, trying to be funny. But there was nothing funny or clownish about it. It was the only way he could walk. Doctors had a term to describe his walk—waddling gait.

In retrospect, I wonder how he was always able to keep a smile on his face. How could a kid who knew that his body was getting weaker every day, who knew that he was taking the last few steps of his life, be the one among us who smiled the most?

Every day his waddle worsened until one day he showed up to school in a push wheelchair.

Although I never gave it much thought at the time, watching Duane struggle during his last days on his feet and being around him during the time when he was forced to come to terms with life in a wheelchair are memories that I would only come to value many years later. Only recently—several years after that chance encounter in 2002 and after actually becoming real friends with him—did it occur to me that I had the pleasure to witness something neither his wife nor his son ever did. I got to see Duane walk.

My Glass is Half Full

In Spring 2011, shortly after I published my first book, *One Way Ticket to Anywhere*, a memoir about the challenges I faced growing up, Duane Hale became my self-appointed, number-one promoter, recommending my book to everyone who would listen. His Facebook posts were persistent. I hadn't seen him in a few years so I invited him to lunch so I could thank him in person.

When I walked into Cracker Barrel, I was taken aback to see his mother, Peggy, feeding him. She lifted a fork of mashed potatoes to her forty-six-year-old son's mouth as she explained why they were already eating. "We went ahead and ordered since it takes so long for Duane to eat."

It made sense, I thought. When one person feeds two mouths it simply takes longer. Later I'd learn another reason it takes my friend longer to eat than most of *us*. Just in the last few years, the disease has begun to affect Duane's ability to swallow his food. After a few close calls, he has learned to chew very carefully. If a potato skin or kernel of corn stalls in his throat on the way down, he doesn't have enough muscle to cough it up.

So then what happens?

Heimlich maneuver?

Nope. Under his button-up shirt, Duane wears a hard plastic brace around his upper body, from his waist to just under his chin.

How do you save a turtle from choking?

It's like a bad joke without a punchline.

The solution is prevention. Duane takes small bites and chews his food very well before swallowing.

Between those small bites he told me that he couldn't drive anymore either. "They took away my keys because I kept running over trashcans."

When I had invited him to lunch I hadn't realized he could no longer feed or drive himself. The last time I saw him, a few years earlier, he could do both.

As his mother raised a fork of brisket toward his mouth, Duane lifted his right forefinger, a cue to his mother to hold on one second. He wanted to finish his thought about how things had been changing in his life. "We used to go out to eat all the time, but…well…the last couple years…I'm having a hard time with people seeing me be fed. I haven't eaten in public for several months."

Clearly, him being out with me was a big deal. Only later would I come to understand just how clueless I was about the logistics and arranging it took to get Duane from his bed to a table at Cracker Barrel.

I had this sudden teenage, high school eating memory of Duane. My group of friends stopping and chatting for a few minutes with his group of friends at the East Texas Fair while they sat at a picnic table. For some unexplained reason, I remembered Duane thirty years before gnawing on a cob of corn he held to his mouth with both hands. That random recollection brought the present into perspective. *Imagine, being forty and having the eating skills of an eight-month-old baby in a high chair. How many messes, spills and drops did he endure before once-and-for-all giving up? How does a man keep from going insane?*

After he finished eating, his head swiveled over his otherwise motionless body as he seemed to scan the dining room for people he recognized. Situated on Interstate 20, at a services-laden exit midway between Shreveport, Louisiana and Dallas, Texas, the majority of these Cracker Barrel diners were travelers, but locals eat there too. I noticed him give a head nod and smile toward a family at a table near us.

"Do you know them?" I asked.

"Nope," he said. "But I noticed the little boy was staring at me."

A minute later, he smiled and said "hello" to a couple that passed by our table.

"Do you know them?"

"I think so. I just can't remember from where. When you live in one place your whole life and work at the police department for twenty years, you've pretty much seen every face in town at least once," he laughed.

During the course of the meal, two ladies came one-by-one to the table to chat with Duane, his mother, and his son. It was like eating lunch with a celebrity.

When we finished eating I walked out to the parking lot with his family and watched his mother deploy the lift from the van. As I watched him rise on the elevator, I got this sense of déjà vu. But it wasn't déjà vu; I was watching a scene from my childhood repeat itself. I was having another sudden-memory-moment of Duane:

I'm leaving school and so is Duane. His mother is raising him on a lift into their van. It was almost as if he were being taken away by a spaceship to another planet only to reappear magically at school the next day.

I remember wondering what Duane's life was like after those van doors closed. What was it like to be him?

After lunch, during my two-hour drive home, I found those questions coming back to me. I not only wondered what his childhood was like after those van doors closed, but I had thirty more years to wonder about. How have his parents coped with the disease? How has he lived in a world built for people like me? What had he really done since we went to high school together? What gave him the strength to get up every day?

I thought Duane to be a fascinating subject. I was impressed how a man could maintain so much dignity even as his son, mother, and wife fed him and helped him perform the most intimate and personal tasks.

The next night I decided to ask him for the privilege of helping him write his story.

"I was hoping you'd ask me that," he said. "I've been wanting to share my story with others for some time."

So began a partnership. I spent many days working with Duane—he in his bed, me in a chair beside it. We talked and I wrote. After a couple of hours I'd get restless. My attention span would wane so I'd head out to my car and run an errand, sometimes visit with an old friend, or maybe just drive around my hometown and contemplate how much things change. I'd come back from my little break and Duane would still be in his bed, in the same position. It occurred to me how much I took everything for granted—my health, mobility, my lifestyle. There are no breaks for Duane.

Although he can no longer feed himself while upright in his wheelchair, when we started writing he could lay at just the right angle in his bed, rest his right elbow on the mattress, grip a cup and lift it to his mouth.

One day, while we were working on this manuscript, I watched him take a drink from his cup. It occurred to me that I was thirsty and wanted a refill of my own drink. I went to the kitchen where Duane's wife, Kim, intercepted me and my empty glass. She poured me a glass of Coke and smiled as I thanked her. Actually, she only poured half a glass before stopping. This was the second time she had filled my glass only halfway. *Hmm, maybe money's tight over here and she's rationing soda.* I went back to Duane's bedside with my half-filled glass of Coke.

A little later Kim joined our conversation about Duane's physical limitations. "He can still drink from an open cup, but because of the angle he's lying, if I fill it too full, he spills it on his chin and runs down his chest."

"Did you know you filled my glass only halfway, too?" I asked.

She started blushing. "I'm so sorry. Every time I pour a drink I only fill it halfway, even mine and Logan's. It's just a habit."

"You know," I said, speaking to both Duane and Kim. "Half full…it's kind of symbolic, isn't it? Duane always seems so positive…so…optimistic."

Duane answered. "A lot of people get diseases where they're in pain all the time. Even though I can't move, at least I'm not always hurting. I have SMA Type

3. If I had Type 1 you would never have known me. If I had Type 2, I probably would've never had Kim or Logan. Think about it Rich, most people in my condition are in a nursing home…alone. I'm with my wife and son every day. If I wanna go out somewhere, my wife or mother takes me. I have a life—people who love me and care for me. Even if I don't make it out of bed, I have a reason to 'get up' every day. When I compare all that to the life I could have, my glass IS half full."

Death Sentence

"It's not all in my head."
--Peggy Hale [to her son's doctor]

His mother was the first to suspect that Duane had problems. Even though he was her first child, Peggy Hale knew her son was not developing strength and dexterity at the same rate as other kids his age. She took her toddler son to several different doctors in Tyler looking for answers. "My little boy is almost two and he's having a hard time walking," she told one doctor.

"He's just flatfooted and knock-kneed," the doctor said.

Months later, she was referred to a specialist who was even less help. "Oh, there's nothing wrong with him. Some boys just develop slower than others."

Peggy knew better. She had watched Duane struggle just to stand up. She knew she was dealing with lazy or incompetent doctors, not a lazy or slow-developing son.

A third doctor was worse than the first two, telling her it was "all in her head."

Peggy was infuriated. Just two weeks before she had watched her son wobble into their family Christmas tree and grab a branch in a futile attempt to regain his balance, first pulling the tree down on top of himself, then sending her into labor with Duane's sister. The combination of taking care of a newborn and another disinterested doctor filled her with about as much Christmas cheer as *The Grinch*. She wasn't going to go away quietly this time. "What do you mean, 'in my head'?"

To prove her point, she walked to the other side of the exam room and called for her two-year-old son to walk toward her. The little boy with fair skin, blonde curly hair, and big brown eyes took a few wobbly steps before his knees buckled and he fell to the seated position. Then he rolled over onto his hands and knees. While kneeling on all fours, like a four-legged animal, he stepped with his right leg and quickly placed his right hand on his right knee. While balancing tenuously on his left knee and right foot, he put his left hand on his left thigh and pushed mainly with his right hand until he reached a crouch. Next, he straightened his legs by inching his hands one-by-one further up his thighs until he reached a traditional Japanese deep bow position. With a final push of each hand against his upper thighs, he raised his upper body to finally stand erect. Then he waddled a few more steps until he fell into his mother's waiting arms.

Peggy looked at the doctor. "My boy is twenty-eight months and he can't even walk ten feet across the room without his legs giving out."

The doctor suggested that she come back in three months if her son was still having trouble walking and standing.

She’d had enough. “If you don’t know what’s wrong just tell me you don’t know, but don’t tell me it’s my imagination. I’ll find a new doctor.”

A succession of doctors appointments in Dallas became family torture rituals and yielded no answers. For two years Duane's mother and father would take off work every few months for the four-hour round trip drive to the big city hospitals. During the first couple of visits the Dallas doctors did nothing that the Tyler doctors hadn't already done.

Duane’s mother recalls how maddening it was to deal with incompetent doctors. "A Tyler doctor takes his temperature, blood pressure, taps his knees with rubber triangles, weighs him and tells me there's nothing wrong.

I asked for a referral to a specialist and he sends me to a doctor in Dallas who does the same thing. How can five different doctors watch a two-year-old’s knees buckle after taking three steps and then simply shrug it off? How can two parents who have never been to college be more astute than pediatricians, orthopedists, and specialists? For years we knew there was something wrong but we couldn't find a doctor smart enough to figure out he had a relatively common disease."

Duane’s case was tossed around like a hot potato, each doctor referring to another or taking a nonchalant, wait-and-see approach.

During one visit to the doctor, six needled probes were jabbed into one of his calves. The wires attached to the probes led to a monitor. The doctor told him to flex his calf. When he did, the graphs on the display squiggled. The doctor thought that was good. "Your son's muscles are reactive," he said. They were sent home with no follow-up appointment.

"We spent a whole day just to learn that Duane's calves cause graphs to squiggle." Peggy recalled. "That put us behind another few months because no one cared that he couldn't walk as long as his muscles made squiggles on paper."

Doctor appointments were usually followed by days of crying. It was almost like a tragic movie plot, but these were real doctors who were either uninformed, apathetic or both, and this was a real family who went years without a diagnosis.

By his fourth birthday, Duane still waddled. Not even the most incompetent doctor could deny there was something not right with a four-year-old boy who wobbles around like a drunk and crawls up staircases. Doctors finally got around to taking Duane's symptoms seriously. "It was such a relief when they started acknowledging that there was a problem," Peggy said. "At least they started trying."

On each visit they conducted useless tests, some of them very invasive. X-rays, scans, physical exams, dyes and other fluid injections, and lab reports yielded no diagnosis. The night after having dyes injected into his spine, he broke out in fever, cold sweats and unbearable joint pain. He was back in Dallas the next day where doctors strapped him onto a table and tilted and rolled him until they added dizziness and nausea to his list of symptoms.

Finally they found a physician who made the right diagnosis. That doctor called Duane's parents into his office. "Mr. and Mrs. Hale, I'm afraid Duane has tested positive for Kugelberg-Welander.

This meant nothing to Peggy and Larry.

"It's a muscle disease," the doctor continued. "A counselor is going to join us in just a minute."

Duane's parents were confused. Information was coming at a slow pace as if the doctor was being paid by the hour.

"A counselor? What do you mean, a counselor?" Larry asked.

The doctor seemed to be stalling, but Larry forced him into starting his medical overview of the disease before the counselor arrived. But this doctor was a poor communicator of details. For some reason he avoided referencing the disease by its more informative and descriptive name, Spinal Muscular Atrophy.

"Kugelberg-Welander is caused by a genetic defect. You need to understand that there is no cure."

The doctor finished, "…because of this defect, his muscles will wither away from lack of use. Duane will likely have a few years of functional strength to perform only basic tasks until the age of about ten. At that point, you can expect he will require a wheelchair to get around. Very few patients diagnosed with this disease at Duane's age make it out of their teenage years."

Peggy began to break down and cry. The words *NO CURE* made it hard to focus on anything else. She buried her head in her husband's chest. Neither could believe what they were hearing.

The counselor entered the conference room, introduced herself and took over. "Mrs. Hale, there are some real strong support groups for families with these diseases."

The doctor had just told her and her husband that their son wouldn't live to see adulthood. The last thing she wanted to hear was some counselor babble about support groups.

The counselor droned on. "Each of you is a carrier of a defective gene. But it's important that you don't blame yourselves."

She looked at the doctor. "What if you're wrong?"

"I wish I was," the doctor said. "Our diagnosis is conclusive"

Duane's parents held little regard for the opinions of doctors. If all the previous physicians were unable to diagnose the disease why should they accept this doctor's prognosis? They had a hunch the medical community still had a lot to learn about their son's disease. Their intuition couldn't have been more correct. To be fair to the medical community, it wouldn't be until a quarter of a century later, in 1995, when researchers would identify the precise SMA-determining gene. Duane's parents had no way of knowing at the time that this doctor was just as misinformed as all the others. They didn't know that there were thousands of people with Duane's disease living into middle age. There was no Internet. There were no alternate resources. There was only one doctor telling them their son had ten or twelve years to live.

Peggy was defiant. "Three different doctors have told me the problem is everything from flat feet to my imagination. Now you're sitting there telling me he's gonna die as a teenager? I don't believe you. That is unacceptable."

The counselor tried to bring her back to reality as gently as possible.

"Mr. and Mrs. Hale, I know this is a hard thing to hear, but you can raise him one of two ways: Either as a *handicapped* child or as a *normal* child. What I mean by that is, you can do everything for him to make his short life comfortable, or you can force him to do as much as possible on his own. You can keep him out of school or you can try to enroll him and see how it goes. It's all up to how the family wants to handle this."

The word *normal* hit Larry especially hard. It was as if the experts were telling them that they could pretend their son is *normal*, even try to fool him into thinking he is *normal*, but that we all know he is not normal. Certainly there was no offense intended in the counselor's word choice. They had recognized long ago that there were certain aspects of their son's development that were not normal, but they never thought of him as anything but a normal person. It almost sounded as if they were being told that there are two kinds of people—normal and freaks—and that all they could do is *pretend* their son is normal.

Larry asked the doctor, "Is there anything we can do? Anything at all that will help?"

"I'm sorry to say, not only is there no cure, but there aren't even any medications that reduce the symptoms or delay the onset. There is only one thing you can do to slow the march of SMA as it pervades Duane's body—force exercise."

"Force exercise?" Larry asked.

"Yes…use it or lose it," the doctor responded.

Or more accurately, use it and lose it later.

The couple was walking out of the doctor's office when Peggy happened to survey the children in the waiting room. It was a heart-wrenching sight. Some kids were hunched over in wheelchairs and couldn't look up. Several had limb deformities. Others seemed to have severe mental retardation. One moaned and drooled on himself.

Even in the face of the devastating news she had just received, Peggy was able to avoid wallowing in self-pity. *I can handle this. I must be positive. Those doctors are always wrong on everything. Duane is better off than all those children, and for that, we are lucky.* It was that kind of positive attitude and perspective that Duane's parents knew they needed to teach him.

They decided that they would push Duane to be as close to normal as possible. Of course they knew there would be limitations, but they wanted him to be somewhat self-reliant. There were things that they knew he could do for himself, and for those things, his parents insisted that he do so.

His father was especially hard on him, challenging Duane to push his physical limits. "Use it or lose it," his father sometimes told Duane. If Larry was going to err, he was going to err on the side of pushing his son too hard, rather than not enough.

Peggy and Larry both believed that the more Duane did for himself, the better his spirit—and in the long run, his health—would be. They weren't going to raise him as a handicapped child. They were going to raise him as a normal child.

It was a conscious decision that wasn't always easy to practice but would ultimately play a role in Duane outliving many of his doctors. It was an attitude Peggy and Larry cultivated in their son who would spend his whole life in a fight to be "normal."

One in Ten Thousand

SMA comes in four numbered flavors—Types 1 through 4. The victim's prognosis improves as the number increases. Type 1 is the most severe. The majority of Type 1 SMA babies present symptoms almost immediately and Type 1'ers account for the fact that **SMA is the most frequent genetic cause of infant mortality**.

Duane has Type 3 SMA. Although Type 3 and the complications resulting from it has taken many young lives long before their time, there are other Type 3'ers with remarkable stories similar to Duane's. Fathering a child and living as long as he has does not make him a freak of nature but it does put him in the minority of Type 3'ers.

About one in fifty people, both men and women, are carriers of the SMA-causing gene. Using basic arithmetic, about one out of every 2500 man/woman unions are between an SMA-carrying man and an SMA-carrying woman. For every birth from a SMA-carrying couple, one out of four will be a child who has the disease, two out of four will be a carrier, and one out of four are unaffected. For those who failed high school algebra, that means the odds of a baby having some type of SMA are about one in ten thousand.

In Duane's lifetime, both prenatal and carrier testing has been developed. Because overall incidences of SMA are "only" one in ten thousand, doctors rarely prescribe any testing unless there is a family history of SMA.

The recent successes in the research, identification, and testing of the SMA-causing gene not only offer us hope but also give us the expectation that, for the one in ten thousand born with SMA there will soon be a cure

Jerry's Kid

Duane

"This is the year. With all those millions of dollars pouring in, how could this not be the year that they find a cure?"
--Duane

Each September, I stayed up as late as I could to watch the Jerry Lewis MDA Labor Day Telethon. My eyes were glued to our console color TV as Jerry called for the tote board to roll every hour.

In my mind, every million-dollar milestone bought more hope for a cure. I remember when they broke the ten-million-dollar mark and Ed McMahon painted a "1" to the left of the other seven digits. The numbers grew each year and every Labor Day I thought, "This is going to be the year of the cure."

The hoopla of the annual event gave me hope to imagine myself as a cured adult. The shows also left my child's mind with the impression that money was the only obstacle to a cure—that if enough people gave enough money I would not only walk again, but one day I'd run and lift heavy things. *If only people gave more money I could help my dad on his farm. I could hoist big bags of feed onto my shoulders and take care of cattle.*

The broadcasts showed clips of scientists mixing up potions in beakers, looking through microscopes, staring at molecular diagrams on chalkboards. I likened the pursuit of a cure to the hardest math problem on a test—one that the whole class got wrong. At one point I even dreamed of becoming a scientist and joining the research team. How cool would that be—to cure my own disease and help the kids at MDA camps all over the world get up from their wheelchairs and walk?

Through my teenage years, around the time I lost my own battle to walk, the combination of my growing awareness and the advancement of the disease chipped away at my hope for a cure. Each telethon seemed like a broken record of the one before. I began to notice there were several clips that were reruns of the previous year. The transformation from *hope* to *acceptance* was a gradual one.

I don't want to sound ungrateful or even cynical about the *Muscular Dystrophy Association* or Jerry Lewis. Both the organization and the man have done so much for our cause. Jerry Lewis worked forty-five years to raise global awareness and over a billion dollars for Muscular Dystrophy. Some of my best childhood moments were at MDA camps that were funded by millions of private individuals and thousands of businesses and corporations.

Researchers funded in part by MDA have now progressed to the cusp of a cure. However, at some point many years ago, I stopped kidding myself. Given my age, I came to accept that there was no chance for me to be cured. So I stopped hoping for myself and adopted a live-for-today mindset. I still have hope—not for myself, but for today's SMA and MD kids and for tomorrow's ALS victims.

The Other Kid In a Wheelchair

In June of 2011, I was having my first bedside brainstorming session with Duane. It had been two weeks since our lunch at Cracker Barrel. He looked so put together that day at the restaurant. He was dressed nice and clean-shaven, sitting perfectly erect in his wheelchair. He sat with the same almost-military-attention posture that I remembered from thirty years before—shoulders square and his chest puffed out.

But on this day—my first day on the job—Duane looked much different. He was lying at a thirty-degree angle in a hospital-style bed. A sheet was pulled up to his chest exposing bare shoulders, but covering the curves of his bent and upward-pointing legs. He smiled as I walked into the room. "Thanks for coming and perfect timing. Would you mind helping me use the toilet?"

He left me hanging for a second or two until his smile gave away the joke.

Within minutes of settling in we were in work mode. He was telling me stories while I feverishly took notes and asked questions.

"Do you remember Billy Brewster?" he asked.

"I didn't know him, but I know about him. I think he passed away while still in high school, didn't he?

Seems like I remember a tribute to him in an old yearbook."

Duane's right elbow rested on the mattress, snug against his ribs, as he swung his lower right arm a few inches, rolled his wrist outward and gripped a cup of water. He slowly lifted the cup to his mouth and took a big drink. Then he methodically lowered it back onto the service tray until one edge of the circular bottom of the cup tapped the surface. He opened his grip slightly and the bottom of the cup went into a small, but noticeable, controlled slide until the cup was resting upright. Then he returned his hand to his stomach—a place that I would later observe to be its usual resting position. "Before me, there was Billy Brewster."

When Duane was in elementary school, he was the "other" kid in town with a muscular disease. Duane's friend was seven years older and had Duchenne Muscular Dystrophy. Billy lived just a few houses away. The two attended fund-raising functions and other social activities together while their families formed a kinship based on their facing similar challenges.

In 1970, the medical community was in the infant stage of differentiating between the muscular diseases and tended to lump them together, delivering a grim prognosis to the parents of the children who had them. Today, we know Billy's Duchenne MD is the most aggressive form of muscular diseases. The doctors who in 1970 told Duane's parents that it was unlikely he'd make it out of his teens didn't understand that although Duane's particular type of SMA ravaged its victim's bodies to the same extent that Duchenne did, it would likely do so at a slower rate.

***

Being tagged by doctors with the same prognosis as Billy meant Duane perceived his older friend's battle against MD as the road ahead of him. For most boys, being seven years younger means being seven years weaker. For kids with degenerative muscular diseases, it's just the opposite. Duane was always more physically-able than his older friend, and watching the effects of the disease progress in Billy left an indelible mark in young Duane's mind.

Several times they appeared together on the local TV affiliate as part of the *Jerry Lewis Labor Day Telethon*. Duane remembers Billy's last appearance on the show. A small group of *Jerry's Kids* sat in their wheelchairs in a lounge area at the studios, watching the telethon feed on TV. A volunteer brought sodas to the kids. Although he wouldn't win any arm wrestling competitions, Duane's arms were fully functional for basic tasks and he drank from his bottle as easily as any kid his age would.

The volunteer had placed Billy's soda bottle on a tray above his lap, about twelve inches from his mouth and then bustled away to attend to other duties. Duane thought nothing of the bottle in front of Billy. His friend had always been able to grip light objects with his dominate right hand and lift them to his face. But that day at the television studio, each time Billy tried to close the grip of his right hand around the soda bottle, it slipped from his fingers and shifted a few inches to the left. He tried about four times until the drink had slid so far that, despite valiant efforts, he could no longer stretch his right arm far enough across the tray to reach it. His drink was situated in a better position for his left arm to handle the chore, but atrophy had taken away Billy's lesser-utilized arm a year or more earlier. Even after someone came by and helped Billy grip the soda bottle, he lifted it to his mouth but was unable to tilt it.

Even as a nine year old, Duane knew that a muscular disease victim's last thread of self-reliance is based on being able to make this movement. If you can loosely grip a light object and lift your hand to your face, you could feed yourself, tend to your own drink, brush away pesky insects, wipe a runny nose, scratch a facial itch, wash your face, adjust glasses, clear sleep from your eyes.

A flood of paralyzing fear came over Duane as he watched Billy struggle with his drink. He froze, not yet with muscle atrophy, but with fear—no more capable of moving at this moment than Billy was. *I'm not just watching Billy. I'm seeing myself in seven years.*

***

A few months after the telethon, Duane was in his bedroom when his mother came into the room. Tears welled in her eyes. "Jimmie Brewster just called—"

Duane knew the rest, but his mother struggled to finish anyway. "Billy passed away." At ten years old, Duane received the news hard. Not only had he lost a friend, but doctors had already told his family that he was on the same course as Billy. Now he had a date. *Seven years.* Peggy Hale hugged her son and left the room to visit with the Brewsters, becoming one of the first visitors to offer condolences in their home.

Duane's role model of how to fight the disease was gone. He was alone in his battle. MD had taken Billy Brewster from his family and from the town of Lindale, and even as he faced his fear that he might be next, Duane Hale began his tenure as the smiling face of perseverance in his community.

When the school yearbook came out, Duane saw the page-one tribute in memory of Billy Brewster who died while a junior in high school. Duane set a goal. Simple and attainable he thought. To make it a year longer than Billy did—to graduate high school.

H-O-R-S-E

There was a time when he got out of bed in the morning, washed, ate breakfast, got dressed, gathered his things, walked to the car, crawled into the backseat with his sister and accessed any building in town he wanted. He didn't play sports, couldn't keep up with his friends and playmates when they ran, and got picked on just a little like any scrawny, weak boy does. Otherwise, at least for a few preteen years, Duane thumbed his nose at SMA. Although his parents managed around his limitations, he didn't require constant care. He was close to *normal,* just as his parents had decided to raise him.

After he reached his physical peak at the age of ten, his walking radius gradually diminished. Some of his favorite places, the playground, the ballfield, the pond, and several of his friends' houses were no longer walking destinations. His world began shrinking.

When Duane was in fourth grade, he could walk for ten minutes without getting tired. His pace was slow—less than a third of the walking speed of his classmates. It took patience to be friends with him. Not all elementary school-aged kids were tolerant enough to wait for Duane.

By fifth grade, Duane was tired of being last in line for everything. One day before lunch, he climbed on Les Melvin's back, wrapped his long right arm around the front of his friend's neck, wedged the inside of his elbow under Les' chin, gripped his friend's left shoulder with his right hand, clutched his own right wrist with his left hand and told his new personal pony to *giddyup*.

Les reached both hands behind his back, grabbed Duane behind his knees, lifted, leaned forward a little and took off running. They both laughed as they zoomed past their classmates arriving at the cafeteria to discover there was no line. They were first! Duane wasn't accustomed to being first. It was a celebratory, light-hearted moment for both of them and they laughed and smiled about the immediate service as the lunch ladies slopped Salisbury steak and peach cobbler into the partitioned squares of their lunch trays. But it was also a profound turning point, one that happens to all SMA kids. Duane realized that his friend's legs could get him around three times as fast as his own. He had found an alternative method. He'd adapted; something most SMA and MD children learn to do better than their able-bodied peers.

After lunch, he hitched a ride on Les' back to the playground. When they got to the basketball court, Les lowered Duane onto his own feet, where they played a game of H-O-R-S-E using a tennis ball. The ten-foot rim was just within range of Duane's underhand tosses. Duane once tried to shoot a basketball. It was so heavy he couldn't get it much above eye level. After a few minutes, a crowd of kids invaded their once-private court with a half-dozen basketballs.

He wasn't looking when one of them rebounded off the rim and clobbered him in the head. Duane stumbled, lost his balance and fell forward.

Imagine you trip in a parking lot and start falling forward. Now suppose your arms are strapped tightly to your sides and ninety percent of the muscle in your legs has been removed. It's hard to even visualize the concept of falling forward without arms, isn't it?

What's going to keep your head from hitting solid concrete?

Your neck muscles?

Oh…I forgot to add that eighty percent of those are gone as well.

Your stomach and chest will hit hard and your head will whiplash into solid pavement. Only with God's grace and good luck would you survive without a serious head injury.

It seems odd to remark that a ten-year-old boy who can't throw a basketball more than one foot above his hands was in the best condition of his life, but Duane was lucky that he was able to twist a little to land primarily on his right shoulder and that his arms worked just enough to slightly cushion the impact and that his neck stiffened just enough to leave only a minor bump on his forehead. Had it happened a year or two later, after Duane's arms had weakened even more, he might have suffered a life-threatening injury.

A few boys laughed. How could they fathom that a seemingly silly moment like a basketball rebounding off a rim and bouncing off someone's head could turn tragic? The danger of a simple fall for MD or SMA children who are still walking is a concept that is hard even for mature adults to comprehend.

Les and a couple of other boys helped him up. Duane waddled off the court and rested his butt against the thick, gray-black, brick fence that surrounded the campus.

"Alright, let's play a game," one of the boys said.

Duane fingered the small bump on his head while watching his friends play basketball. They were oblivious to the fact that they'd not only run him off the court that he was playing on first but they also narrowly missed putting him in the hospital. They weren't being mean; they just didn't know any better. When the playground monitor, Coach Daniels, blew the whistle signifying the end of lunch recess, Duane rode Les to their next class.

From that day forward, Duane knew the most practical way of getting around at school would be to ride on the strong backs of his friends. Over the next couple of years, a few others took turns lugging him around campus. Although they all seemed to enjoy helping, none of them would log the kind of heavy mileage Les did.

The Leader of the Band

"His own disease causes his head to tilt downward. It's like he was genetically engineered to look straight into my eyes as I sat in my wheelchair."
--Duane [on Butch Almany]

Duane

If you grow up in the mountains of Colorado, you probably want to be a skier. If you grow up on the beach in Hawaii, you might dream of being a surfer. If you grow up in Lindale, the only thing that rivals being on the football team is to be in the Lindale High School Marching Band. The passion for both football and band was so ingrained in Lindale's culture that it was almost impossible to register on the social radar unless you were involved in at least one of the two.

I certainly couldn't play football so I always dreamed of being in the band.

I spent a good part of my childhood watching my friends compete. In first and second grade, I tried to get involved in some of playground games but I just couldn't keep up. I gave kickball a shot, but when it was my turn to kick, I couldn't even kick the red, rubber ball back to the pitcher. Even if I could have kicked, I sure couldn't run afterward.

I wasn't able to throw any ball, except a tennis ball, more than a couple feet. So I spent school recess playing marbles and *Hot Wheels* under the big oak tree on the edge of the playground. Depending upon what else was happening, I might waddle over to watch my friends play football or basketball. For the most part I felt like Rudolph—excluded from the reindeer games.

Most boys were pretty focused on physical games, but every once in a while, Eric Bartley or Cary Johnson would come over and play marbles with me or just talk for a while.

One day, a new kid came over and started talking to me. "Hey, can I see your Hot Wheels?"

"Sure." I said. "My name's Duane."

"Mine's Ronald Bunch."

A few days later, while everyone else was playing tag football, Ronald had me hold a plastic bat while he pitched me tennis balls. I gave a few weak swings but couldn't make contact with the ball. Finally, Ronald had me hold the bat out while he threw. After about ten tries, the ball hit the bat that I was holding and dribbled out a few feet in front of me. That was the closest I'd ever come to hitting a home run.

I wanted to compete in something. Even if it wasn't athletics, I wanted to be in contests to measure myself against others in something. I wanted to be part of some kind of team or unit. I'd never joined any organized group or competed in anything. That would all change in sixth grade.

In those days, nearly half the student body played in the band. For twenty-four years, the architect of the band's success and popularity was its director, Butch Almany.

I wanted to be in that band, which meant I was eager to join the intermediate school band at the earliest opportunity—sixth grade. My parents didn't make a lot of money. Although medical bills, wheelchairs, lifts, van, and all my other disease stuff had already put a financial strain on the family, my parents worked overtime and set money aside. In August, just before sixth grade, they bought me a cornet for my eleventh birthday. The instrument represented their approval and commitment to support me in joining the band. I chose the cornet mainly because it was light and easy to handle.

For a month before school started, I struggled first just to make a sound with my new instrument, then to play a note. I practiced simply holding the horn to my mouth for several minutes at a time.

On the first day of sixth grade, I carried my new cornet that I had no idea how to play into the band hall of one of the most iconic educators to ever grace my town. I hoped things that I'd heard about Mr. Almany were true. Could a man really take a kid with nothing but ambition—a kid who could barely get his instrument to make a noise—and train him how to play beautiful music? Would he really bring out the best in me, like everyone said he did for his students?

I wasn't sure if I had the wind or the arm strength that it took to play an instrument, let alone any musical talent.

• • •

I heard Mr. Almany was tough on his students, that he was a perfectionist. Rumor had it that he only taught sixth grade because he wanted to weed out the underachievers before they got to high school. Several older kids told me he tended to call people out individually in front of the whole band. I feared I'd be one of those people—that I would be the first one. I imagined him stopping down in the middle of our very first practice to humiliate me. I could picture it in my mind. "Stop! Stop! Duane Hale, is that you making that God-awful racket? Go to the office and tell them I said to put you in study hall because your cornet is hurting my ears. I can't have that noise in my band." I worried my band experiment would have a humiliating end. Would it be the same as me trying to kick a ball? Would I lag behind in band just as I had on the playground?

Within weeks, I was at ease. Although he never seemed to treat me any different than anyone else, the fact that Mr. Almany was also a frail cornet player with a degenerative disease, Anklyosing Spondilitis (AS), might have made him sensitive to my condition. His AS, which is an arthritic disease, caused him to walk with a gimp. But more than that, it contorted his body toward a forward lean and a downward tilt to his head. Because of his lean and head tilt, Mr. Almany, like me, also looked up at the world. To me, his posture made him appear inviting because he leaned toward people during conversation, almost like he was bending in to hear a secret.

I was amazed at how fast I learned to play. It was one of the most exciting learning experiences of my life. He pushed me, like he pushed everyone. He had an amazing ear. I quickly learned there was no fooling Mr. Almany. I couldn't claim to have practiced a piece when I hadn't. He always knew. He had this aura about him that made us students not want to be the one to disappoint him. You wanted to please Mr. Almany. You want him to approve of your sound.

Mr. Almany's high school bands received Sweepstakes awards twenty consecutive years. They played for the President and for the Governor of Texas. They were the pride of Lindale. When I started in sixth grade I hoped that I would be good enough three years later to play for him again in the Lindale High School Marching Band.

When I went into my wheelchair, I realized our diseases brought us a unique point-of-view of each other—one that nobody else shared. Ironically, the combinations of our conditions brought us eye-to-eye in the physical sense. Of all the people he dealt with, only my eyes landed in is natural line of sight. Mr. Almany's head tilt was humble, yet his gaze was intimidating. Because of his posture I had the unique experience of connecting with him eye-to-eye more than anyone else. I was the only person he could talk to whom he didn't have to look up at. In the physical sense, and as a mentor, Mr. Almany had me in his sights.

In high school, Mr. Almany encouraged me to join his prestigious stage band. My parents came through again, this time buying me a shiny, silver trumpet. By then I needed to raise the support arms on my wheelchair so I could rest my elbows and forearms on them while I held my trumpet.

After one of my performance solos, he nicknamed me "iceman" because he said I was so cool and collected on stage.

During our stage band rehearsals, Mr. Almany made a few jokes about how hidden I was from the audience's perspective in my wheelchair. "Iceman, I think we're going to have to start calling you "Invisible man." I can't see you. You better make sure I can hear you or I'm counting you absent."

Not that I ever complained, but it did bum me out to know that my face was two feet below the other trumpets in my row, and the woodwind section hid almost my whole body from the crowd. I was proud of being in the stage band and I wanted people to see me.

When I showed up in the auditorium before our first performance for our high school classmates, Mr. Almany greeted me with a smile. "Hey Duane, follow me, please."

He gimped unevenly toward the stage as I wheeled behind him. He glanced me a smile as he pointed to a square wooden riser sitting on the stage, about two feet high with a ramp leading up to it. There was gray skirting around the front of the platform. It was a stage on a stage. He pointed at the ramp. "Can you wheel up to the platform and see if you fit?"

It took me a moment to figure it out; then I realized. Mr. Almany had a platform built for me. That ramp became part of our regular stage rigging and at our concerts my head would be at the same level as the other trumpets. To the audience, I would appear the same height as everybody else.

Mr. Almany put music in my soul and made me feel like a rockstar in his stage band. Mr. Almany quenched that childhood yearning to belong to a team.

The Last Time

"This will be the last time we will ever..."

We say those words when we want to conjure emotion in those we're speaking to. Maybe we hope they will relish *the last time*—cherish it, and hold the moment close to their hearts. Perhaps what we are really trying to do is to help them stamp something permanently into their memories in the same way we are making an effort to burn it into our own.

A football coach tries to inspire his team before their last game of the season. He looks around the locker room and gives a pep talk. "You seniors...for most of you, this is the last time you will strap on shoulder pads and play this game."

A few eighteen-year-old boys look at one another and silently contemplate their lives without football.

The coach finishes. "Now get out there and HIT somebody!"

Duane's life has been, and will continue to be, a series of unceremonious *last times*.

No coach ever slapped him encouragingly on the butt and yelled. "Duane, this is the last time you will ever shower on your own. Now get in there and make it count! And don't forget to wash your feet!" Nor has anyone ever raised a glass and toasted, "Cheers to Duane. This is the last time you will ever walk."

He never could ride a bike, run, do a sit-up, hang from the monkey bars, lift a gallon of milk or raise his legs high enough to climb stairs. For some things, he never had a *first time*, however, other than a few strength-demanding activities he was an active preteen. Unless you happened to see him crawling up or down stairs at seven years old, all you noticed different about him was his walk. But for all the things he could do at eight, most of them he has now already done for the *last time*.

His *last times* are subtle and more private than ours. He senses when a *last time* is creeping up on him. He can feel it as the task becomes exceedingly difficult. But SMA gives him a transition period in task performance. The evolution from *can* to *can't* is often so gradual that the *last time* becomes gray, almost indefinable as a single event.

During those can-to-can't transition phases, Duane's disease forces him to think out of the box. *How can I find an alternative way to do something?* In the case of walking, the new, easier, faster way was to ride piggyback whenever possible.

The day he beat all his classmates to the lunch line marked the beginning of the end of Duane walking. That romp to the school cafeteria began a three-year transition from walking to wheelchair.

Over the course of the next three years, almost through the end of junior high, Les, Neal Mosely, and a few other friends would carry Duane more miles than his own legs.

By eighth grade, he could still take a few steps, but his own legs were no longer a functional method of transportation except to travel short distances. He might waddle within a classroom or in his home but to get around at school, he usually relied on Les and Ronald. In his house, he braced his hands against the walls as he walked, leaving trails of worn drywall and discolored paint in his wake.

The preteen Duane was aware that there were certain things he would never do unless he did them as a child. When he was eleven, he crawled into the attic and walked across the rafters exploring the vents, ducts, plumbing, electrical, and insulation, just so he would know what an attic looked like.

When he was twelve, fearing that he'd never drive unless he made it happen right then, he duct-taped the end of a broomstick to the brake of the family car and with the driver's seat shifted fully forward, took a low-speed joyride around the block.

He was maturing and getting heavier, which meant he was harder to carry. Not only were his legs getting weaker, but they were also being asked to carry more weight. He felt his upper body weakening as well, making it more difficult for him to hold on during piggyback rides.

Three years after that first school piggyback ride, he walked with his wobbly, waddling gait through the school halls under his own power for the *last time*, until his knees buckled and he fell down in the corridor in a heap of crumpled arms and legs for the *last time*.

Two classmates hurried over and carried him to his next class like they were helping a wounded soldier hobble off the battlefield toward a chopper, the boys flanking him on each side, their shoulders lifting his armpits to relieve him of his body weight.

After school, Les carried him piggyback to his mother's waiting car for the *last time.*

He was going to start high school soon and it was time for the next stage of Duane's life to begin. The next day, he showed up for class in a manually-operated wheelchair for the *first time*.

Kids who had carried Duane on their backs immediately became his wheelchair pushers. When he first got the chair, he was all the rage on campus. He let his pushers pop wheelies and build makeshift ramps. Kids took turns pushing his wheelchair into Evel Knievel-style crashes.

As if horseplay wasn't a big enough threat to the integrity of his chair, the junior high school had the most ill-conceived wheelchair ramp in the history of the world. The ten-foot concrete ramp between the playground and the school was around forty-five degrees. One day Ronald slipped while trying to ease Duane's chair down that ramp. When the runaway chair hit the ground, both wheels collapsed sending shrapnel and snapped spokes bending in every direction imaginable and giving Larry Hale his first assignment as his son's wheelchair mechanic.

He was twelve when his parents got him that self-powered wheelchair. They hoped their son would squeeze two or three years out of it. Their hope was that by making him wheel himself around he'd exercise his muscles and help hold back the tide of atrophy invading his shoulders and arms. But unless someone was pushing him, Duane's rolling pace in the manual wheelchair was still too slow to keep up with his peers.

At thirteen, about a year after getting his manually-operated wheelchair, he propelled himself in it for the *last time*. It was time for an electric wheelchair.

At fourteen, his back and stomach muscles were no longer strong enough to hold his growing frame erect in his new wheelchair. In ninth grade, he began to slouch as he struggled to sit upright in his chair. Doctors detected early stage scoliosis, which unaddressed would lead to respiratory ailments and other life-shortening complications.

To prevent rapid progression of scoliosis, Duane had three options: Spend the rest of his life in bed, have a rod surgically implanted into his back, or start wearing a torso brace.

Quitting school to watch TV was not an option. Especially in those days, all they had on daytime TV were soaps. Patients with muscle diseases have a host of increased respiratory risks under general anesthesia. The procedure to insert a rod into Duane's back would be quite invasive. The most practical option was for Duane to start wearing a "turtle shell."

The hard, white, plastic case extends from just under his chin all the way down to his waist. The shell literally holds Duane together so he can sit upright. Without it, his upper body would topple over in his wheelchair like a ragdoll's. No matter how positive his attitude, no matter how strong his spirit, moving to the wheelchair and then into the brace within a year meant that he did a lot of things for the last time.

By fifteen, his legs had become totally useless, shriveled muscle and bone that his caregivers had to bend, straighten, push and tug into place.

In his upper body, the atrophy in his core muscles continued their march slowly outward down his arms. During his teenage years, both of his arms worked pretty well. Through high school, even though his shoulders and arms were weakening, they remained just strong enough to hold his trumpet to his mouth as his elbows rested on his wheelchair armrests. His arms and lungs stayed strong enough to briefly make first chair cornet in the band.

The atrophy crept slowly throughout his twenties down his biceps and triceps and through his forearms. His right arm fought harder and resisted the disease longer, but his lesser-used left arm couldn't keep up.

In his thirties, the range-of-motion and strength of his right arm diminished as those muscles succumbed in the same sequence and fashion, albeit ten years later, as his left side muscles had.

***

Nowadays, Duane can turn his head slightly, breathe, drink, chew his food, talk, and push buttons on a phone or TV remote. He can also push the joystick on his wheelchair. One-by-one those things will be lost.

Every task, every act, every movement that Duane once did is something he has either already lost or is currently in the process of losing. Duane has lived a lifetime of a thousand *I-used-tos*. Each one divides Duane's life into a thousand *befores* and *afters*.

He and I were working together one day on this book. I was in a chair next to him in his bed. We were talking about the range of motion of his right hand. He held his TV remote in his right hand and was using it to rub around his right eye socket.

"See how I'm scratching my eye right now?"

"Yeah…with the remote?" I replied.

"I can't reach my eyes anymore. Just three or four years ago, I could adjust my glasses. Pretty soon, I'm gonna need a longer remote."

If Duane were an element on the periodic table, his half-life would be about six years. At any point in his life, one could compare Duane to what he was six years before and arrive at the conclusion that he can do about half.

Pick any person. Watch them for a few hours. Notice how they scratch their ear, rub their forehead, run a hand through their hair, cover their mouth when they yawn, sneeze or cough. Watch them prepare to eat and wipe their face with a napkin. These subtle face-tending actions are things Duane used to do and all of them are things he once did for *the last time*.

Girls

"Acting like I was trying to run girls over with my wheelchair might've made them laugh, but it didn't help me get any dates."
--Duane

Although being in the band helped give Duane a sense of inclusion, there were other teenage things he was missing out on. He sought a different kind of belonging. Like most other teenage boys, he was interested in girls.

Duane's junior high technique of playfully chasing girls and acting like he was going to run them over with his wheelchair proved to be a less-than-effective courting ritual with the upperclassmen.

During his junior year, he managed to land a girlfriend. Claire was two years younger. The relationship was another connection to normalcy. Like being in the band, it was another way he was like his classmates rather than unlike them. Except for the fact that he needed his parents to chauffeur him on dates, the relationship was a typical high school romance, except he carried her books to class on his wheelchair table.

After a year of going to school dances, sporting events, and hanging out together, and as Duane got closer to graduation, the two had a discussions about the future. The topic of Duane's health was unavoidable. Claire asked questions of Duane that he couldn't answer.

Would he be able to go to college? Would he be able to get a job? If so, what kind of job? How long did he expect to live? Five years? Fifteen? Twenty?

For every question Claire asked, Duane had questions of himself. Would he make enough money to buy a home? Would he ever be able to drive a van without having use of his legs? If so, how would he be able to afford that kind of van?

Duane didn't know the answers to any of those questions. It's not like he never thought about those things, but his spirits were highest when he didn't obsess about his future. He was happiest when he took things one day at a time rather than fret about the progression of his SMA. He didn't like to dwell on the constraints the disease would place on his future.

Duane got a sense that Claire's parents were less than thrilled with their daughter's relationship with him. "I understood the reasons why her parents might be concerned. What parents of a teenage girl dream of their daughter finding a nice boy in a wheelchair who has a paralyzing disease? I never had discussions with them about it, but I'm sure they were worried about their daughter getting hurt. Sensing and understanding the parental influence on Claire's thought process didn't make it any easier on my emotions either of the three times Claire told me she wanted to break up."

Just before graduation, Duane came to terms with the facts. Claire had two more years of high school left and he was moving on from the built-in culture that enabled the relationship. No high school girl wants to be driven to her prom by her boyfriend's parents and then not be able to dance with her date after they get there. Claire needed to experience her last two years of high school without him following her around like some kind of lap dog.

The hardest part of that breakup was the fear that his disease would keep him from ever getting a chance to experience a fulfilling relationship with a girl. Along with all the other things SMA took from him, it also shattered his confidence with the ladies.

Graduation

I wish Brother David Wilkerson were still alive to read this book.
--Duane

The doctor who predicted a teenage death would have been shocked to see Duane twelve years later when his stage band performed at a school assembly. Duane zipped up to center stage in his wheelchair and performed a rousing trumpet solo that brought down the house. Duane realized his disease wasn't going to take him at seventeen. Doctors had told him that his lung capacity and respiratory system were on par with healthy teenagers.

He now expected to graduate high school but took nothing beyond that for granted. Duane had no expectations of going to college but he decided to get the most of his education by making the best grades he could during his senior year of high school.

Counselors had advised his parents that goal setting was important to the emotional health of their son and Duane frequently took the initiative. The goal-setting approach was a mindset that would serve him well for the rest of his life. The focus for his senior year wasn't to win a seat in college or scholarship money or grants. It was simply to make the best grades he could.

He was competing against himself. With every cycle of report cards, he was proud of his grades; they were better than he'd ever scored, but other than his parents, no one seemed to notice. He didn't care. His grades mattered to him even if they didn't matter to anyone else.

During January of his senior year, Duane was called to the office for a meeting with the principal, Elton Caldwell. He told Duane that the Lindale Rotary Club had selected him as *Student of the Month*. He was proud and happy that his hard work was indeed being noticed. He attended a luncheon, got his picture in the paper and his name on a plaque, and was motivated to study even harder for the rest of the school year. He thought about how his goals had changed. Once, all he wanted was simply to live long enough to graduate, now he wanted to graduate with honors.

***

Duane

When I finished junior high, although I relied on my chair for mobility, I was still able to stand and take a few steps. I thought about Billy often through the years, especially as I neared the age at which he died. Relative to Billy, and his battle against Duchenne, I was lucky. As debilitating as SMA was, it was shutting down my body much slower than Duchenne did Billy's. Before my senior year, I set my sights on a more lofty ambition than just to graduate. I wanted to graduate in the top twelve, which would mean special recognition at commencement.

I made straight A's as a senior, but since I had my share of B's in my first two years of high school, it was a little too late to crack the senior top twelve, but I made a good run at it, finishing fifteenth. However, if one measured my academic performance based only on our senior year, I was near the top, and when I put the gown on before the commencement exercise, I knew I had achieved the same standards as my classmates. I was proud to wear my silky, white, National Honor Society cloth around my neck.

During our commencement, a few awards were given. Several students were recognized for their achievements and then the president of the Rotary Club, Kenneth James, whom I'd known for years, stood at the podium to present another award. There was the expected talk about excelling in the classroom, being a model citizen and those types of things. He spoke about the mission of the Rotary Club to provide humanitarian service, encourage high ethical standards in all vocations, and help build goodwill and peace in the world. Mr. James continued. "No one in the Lindale Class of '83 exemplifies the values of the Rotary Club more than the Lindale Rotary Club Student of the Year, Duane Hale."

My heart thumped into overdrive and my body went numb. So many of my classmates had higher grades and were model citizens. *Why did they select me?* As I wheeled up toward Mr. James to receive the award, the applause grew to something more. When I reached the podium, I turned to look at my classmates. They were all standing. I scanned their one-hundred faces and saw one hundred friends. A raging river of memories flooded my mind.

There was Les Melvin who years before acted as my legs.

I saw the big, toothy smile of Henry Williams, who two years prior had come upon me and my stalled chair in the middle of Highway 69. As cars zoomed by, he pushed me to safety.

I caught a glimpse of Kelli McGonagill, the drum major and the leader of our marching band. A year before, while on a band road trip, she and Karen Dickerson brought the *Outstanding Band of Festival* trophy we had won to my hotel room. I remember how excited we all were. "Look what we won Duane!" Kelli said as she extended the five-foot statue toward me as though she expected me to grab it and support its weight. Those girls made me feel as if I'd won the trophy on my own. I knew I'd never forget that moment of hugs, trophies, smiles, and laughter.

Seeing Ronald Bunch's face stirred the deepest emotions of any of my classmates. Since becoming a father at sixteen, he had given up all school-related extra-curricular activities, yet he still found time to care for me. It had become part of his identity. Ronald Bunch—"that guy that's always with Duane." It seemed like only yesterday when he acted like I had hit a ball with my bat when we both knew it was really a case of him hitting my bat with the ball. I wondered how many hundreds of miles Ronald had pushed me over the years. I knew our friendship would endure beyond the halls of a school building.

I also thought about Billy Brewster and how close he came to graduating. I remembered the day he passed and how I set a simple goal to reach this moment.

I looked into the stands and saw my parents, my sister, Sandra, my friends, my town. Every one of them was clapping, cheering, and smiling. I was getting a standing ovation from nearly one thousand people. The irony of the custom of the standing ovation as it relates to my condition hit me. The people who saw me lose my struggle to walk, who had been such a big part of my journey were all expressing their respect, admiration, sympathy, or whatever emotion was inside them, by engaging in a simple ritual—rising from their chairs to stand. As the object of the standing ovation, I was the only one in the gym who was unable to stand. I wondered if anyone else in the gym made the same correlation to the symbolism that I had. The community of Lindale was standing for me because I could not.

A community that had always given so much strength to me in my fight against my disease was now giving me one of the greatest moments of my life. I wanted so much to respond to them in the same way they were acknowledging me. I wanted to stand up just one more time in my life. I wished I could rise from my chair, stand up, just for five seconds, and inspire them in the same way they were inspiring me. I thought about it; wondered if it were possible. Would God and adrenaline give me strength to perform the simple task of supporting my weight with my legs? I had a conversation inside my head as if it were taking place between two people. It would be the last time I ever considered the notion of standing up:

When was the last time I stood for a few seconds?
Three years ago?
Could I do it?

No, don't be ridiculous. Enjoy this moment for what it is. Do not try to be a hero and stand up and break a leg or fall on your face. A trip to the emergency room would ruin this moment.

So I didn't try to stand. And, I knew I would never stand again.

***

I didn't "walk the stage." I wheeled across it and into adulthood. There was no time for me to bask in the moment. Waiting on the other side of that diploma were serious adult issues that demanded my immediate attention.

Out in the crowded foyer, it seemed everyone wanted to take a picture with me. After I posed for what seemed like a hundred shots, a classmate's father approached me. The distinguished man had introduced himself before and had always made it a point to chat with me at school events. "Duane, may I speak to you in private for just one minute?"

I didn't know the man very well, so I wondered why he wanted privacy. "Sure."

We found a semi-private area of the foyer.

Brother David Wilkerson was a world-renowned minister known for his knack for touching the hearts of the hardest of criminals. He had authored many best-selling Christian books, including one that became a movie that has been seen by over fifty million people.

His full head of puffy brown hair was parted on the left and his suit was remarkably crisp. "Duane, we are so proud of you. I am so proud of you." His big strong hand engulfed mine in a handshake.

Having been in a wheelchair for four years, and being a short kid anyway back in the days when I could stand, I was accustomed to people looking down toward me during conversations. But this was different. His elevated physical status didn't seem coincidental; it felt appropriate, as if it were earned by his lifetime of service to God and humankind.

I noticed how engaging his eyes were as he spoke to me. "Duane, that scholarship you won tonight for *Student of the Year* is a nice start, but two-thousand dollars won't even begin to cover all your school needs. I will pay for your college education to any Texas school you want to attend. Here's my card." The hand extending the fancy business card was attached to Brother David Wilkerson, but I felt like I was receiving it from the hand of God. "Duane, you are an inspiration to my son, your whole class, and to me. If you want to go to college, don't worry about the money. I'll take care of it."

A man who is frequently described as an "inspirational leader", was telling me **I** inspired **him**.

I didn't know how to respond other than to humbly thank him.

David Wilkerson, a man whose ministries from Lindale to Times Square are credited with converting thousands of addicts and criminals into Christians and good citizens and a man whose sermons have been heard by untold millions, on the night of his own son's graduation, had his sights set on helping me.

• • •

He gave me a firm man-grip on my shoulder and nodded his approval. "I'll be expecting your call."

I joined my small circle of family and friends. They didn't even notice my two-minute absence.

I can't describe the range of emotions that night: Standing ovations, scholarships, the sense of accomplishment for achieving my goal, thoughts of Billy, the pride I saw in my parents' faces, the definitive end of my relationship with Claire. All those things tugged my heart in different directions. On top of all that, I knew I had reached the end of something good. School was always a safe place for me. Friends, teachers, and the community made it so.

Graduation meant I was no longer the **kid** in a wheelchair; it meant I was the **man** in the wheelchair and I wasn't so sure the world was going to open its arms to a man in the same way it did to a boy.

Now What?

"If I had known I would live this long, I would have gone to college."
--Duane

While all his friends went off to graduation parties, Duane went home. The only party he really wanted to go to was not wheelchair accessible. Claire made an unexpected visit, showing up at his front door, wanting to talk. She was crying. "Maybe, I made a mistake," she said. "Maybe, we should stay together?"

As much as he wanted to agree, Duane knew Claire wasn't really committed. She had attended the commencement and he figured that she was caught up in the emotion of the event.

The phone breakup a week before was fresh in his mind. "I'm concerned about our different life spans," she said just a few days prior. It was an honest comment, and also a valid one, but nonetheless it was a sobering reminder that this was a teenage girl who, just like Duane, wanted her life to be normal.

Her halfhearted suggestion of reconciliation wasn't going to change anything. The relationship had evolved to a place where Duane's disease was becoming the focal point.

SMA had conditioned him to confront reality. Duane didn't have a choice of whether or not to deal with the disease's implications. Claire did. He was devastated by her "lifespan" remark, but at the same time, he understood her concerns. She had been making them clear for several months. Yet there she was, cracking the door open, inviting him to wheel through and reconcile. However, he knew that holding on was futile and for him to do so would be a disservice to both of them and only delay the inevitable.

An hour after a gymnasium full of people stood cheering for him, a half hour after he was offered a full ride to college, he manned up and cleared the conscious of a sixteen-year-old girl, setting her free with the knowledge that the breakup was a mutual decision, even taking accountability for it himself. He didn't want a young girl to feel that she had abandoned a disabled person. He hoped that this last visit, on the night of his graduation, would help Claire to move on without that kind of guilt.

His only high school relationship taught Duane that it would take a unique woman to accept a man with SMA: A selfless yet strong personality that could make up her own mind and be willing to make monumental sacrifices for the sake of love. A woman who wouldn't be influenced by family or friends when they gave her those inevitable I-just-don't-want-you-to-get-hurt speeches.

Duane knew that kind of woman was rare. He wondered if finding such a woman was even possible.

***

In high school, it was cool to be known as Duane's friend. Classmates had often asked to be dismissed from class five minutes early so they could carry Duane's books and open doors for him. Popularity was a function of being a high school student in a small community. The moment he graduated, the concept of popularity was instantly gone. He was no longer the center of attention; he was just some guy in a wheelchair living with his parents.

For as long as he could remember he had been surrounded by hundreds of friends and faculty who went out of their way to accommodate his needs. Soon his beloved band would play without the sound of his trumpet. The cheerleaders who had always clamored to take pictures with him were moving on with their lives. His teachers would have a new crop of students with new needs.

Echoes from his standing ovation the night before still rang in his head as he was already beginning the process of coming to terms with how unpractical, even selfish, it would be for him to attend college. Even with the financial constraints removed and with all the outpouring of emotional support, Duane knew there were too many seemingly insurmountable obstacles to his attending college.

***

Duane

College wouldn't be like high school where I'd been surrounded by a hundred friends on the same schedule.

Maybe if there were a university just around the corner and a bunch of my friends were going, I might be able to work out rides to a couple of classes. But the nearest college campus was twenty miles away and wasn't very wheelchair accessible. Even if it were, who'd drive me back and forth to school? My folks had jobs and I couldn't drive myself. I knew my mother made all kinds of sacrifices above and beyond those she already made if I told her that I wanted to go to college and that Brother Wilkerson wanted to pay for it. How could I impose any more than I already had?

For eight years, I had benchmarked my health against Billy's legacy. Graduation meant I had already outlived my childhood friend by a year and I didn't have any idea of the rate at which my disease would progress. I didn't want to spend what might be the last four years of my life imposing on all who were close to me just so I could have a degree listed in my obituary.

Even if I had stayed strong enough to graduate, what would I do with a degree? What kind of work could I do? In retrospect, I admit that I had somewhat of a defeatist attitude about higher education. I remember thinking, "Who's gonna hire a man in a wheelchair whose condition would only worsen with time?"

I had never used my condition as an excuse to shy away from challenges. I knew I'd done things that no one had expected me to do. But on the matter of college, it seemed to present a lot more obstacles than payoff. I decided that no direction was a better choice than an unrealistic one. My parents would not know of David

Wilkerson's offer until twenty-eight years later when my mother proofread this book just before the first printing—six months too late to thank the man who offered to send her son to college.

I thought about the two thousand dollar scholarship and how it would be wasted. *They should have given that award to someone else, someone who could actually put the scholarship to good use.*

I envied the opportunities that my classmates had and didn't understand why so many of them passed on the chance to pursue a college degree. I would've loved to be in their shoes—to have the choice of being able to go to college.

The morning after that standing ovation at my graduation ceremony, I lie in bed, staring at the ceiling, contemplating my future that would not include college.

Now what?

I Wish I Was Ten Again

The end of high school is a transition for everyone, but Duane's transition was more abrupt. While his friends started college and careers, made new friends, enjoyed their freedom and began their journeys into adulthood, Duane did nothing. His transition was a different one. His whole social network came to a screeching halt. He was no longer one of Jerry's kids. He was a grownup. Even though he was an adult, he felt like he had as a kid at recess—excluded.

His parents had jobs and his sister went back to school in September while Duane hung around the house and neighborhood without structure or direction. Overnight, Duane Hale had gone from the most recognizable and one of the most admired kids in school, to spending most of his day at home alone. He had no structure planned for his days, but he got out of bed out of habit even if he had no specific reason for doing so.

Sometimes he'd drive his chair downtown just to get a soda. It was only a ten-minute trip, but the errand got him out of the house and gave him at least some sense of being a part of the community. The purpose of the outing wasn't about getting a soda. It was a chance of social interaction that prompted the outing. Each trip was filled with hope that he'd run into one or two friends who would take time to stop and chat. Sometimes he'd roll into the bank just for a quick visit with his mother and her co-workers. On a good day, he might run into someone who wanted to sit and have a cup of coffee with him. Sometimes he returned home after not having visited with anyone.

It was during these just-to-get-out-of-the-house excursions that Duane began to understand just how busy and fast-paced the rest of the world was. When he ran into good friends, they didn't always stop to chat very long. A conversation at Smith's Drugstore with a close friend that he hoped might last ten or fifteen minutes often lasted one. His friends weren't rude or aloof. It was a good one-minute; it just wasn't long enough. He started hearing "I'm running late for work, Duane" or "my wife's out in the car waiting for me."

Wait. Don't leave so fast. Don't you understand? This is the high point of my day.

***

Duane

Almost immediately after I finished high school, I started sinking into depression. As if the physical limitations weren't bad enough, the social aspects of the disease contributed to my feelings of isolation. A few years back I could do almost everything my friends did. I just did it at a slower pace.

For the first time in my life, I wasn't busy. The lack of planned activities and any sort of schedule left me feeling without a purpose. I spent a lot of my idle time musing about my childhood. When I encountered old friends around town, I noticed I spent more time reminiscing than I did moving those relationships forward.

When I saw my childhood friends, Karen Dickerson and her sister Cassie Dickerson, at Dairy Queen, we chatted about the long summer days hanging out together with my sister at each other's houses and swimming in our pool and how we caught bees in plastic sandwich bags. We tied thread around their back legs and flew them around like kites. Instead of making plans to do something with them, all we did was talk about things we had done.

I ran into two buddies at Brookshire's. They were stocking up on food for a Fourth of July outing on their boat. We stood/sat in the aisle for twenty minutes and reminisced about climbing trees and playing in the dirt piles near my house. "Let's get together soon, Duane. Let's go do something," one of them said.

"Yeah. Let's do that. Ya'll have a good time at the lake."

For me the romance of those childhood memories was, and still is, more intense than for most people. That was a time when I **looked** and **acted** like everyone else—a time when I was closest to **being** like everyone else. How many nineteen year olds wish they were ten again?

My nineteenth year was probably the hardest of my life. I noticed what was going on around me and it occurred to me that, especially for boys my age, physical activities enhanced friendships. My friends who once popped caps with hammers and caught grasshoppers with me had moved on to playing golf and tennis, hunting, waterskiing, and dirt bike riding. They worked on farms and worked out at the gym while I mostly watched TV. I realized the feelings of isolation were in large part as a result of no longer being able to share activities with my friends. Maybe a nineteen-year-old girl could go shopping at the mall or get her hair and nails done with friends. But I'm a guy, and guys are supposed to do things with their muscles. I wanted to work on a farm with my dad. I wanted to haul hay with my buddies.

My body was heavier and limper than it had been just a few years before. I couldn't ride on my friend's backs anymore. Even the simple act of getting into a friend's car and cruising to Tyler was impractical.

If I wanted to venture beyond a half mile from my house I needed my mom or dad to load me into the van and drive. I relied too much on my parents to connect me to the outside world. While my friends were enjoying their newfound adult independence, I had to ask my mom if she'd take me to the football game. They were growing independent while I was becoming more dependent.

Friends grew stronger while I grew weaker. They formed new relationships. Reduced to soda runs and football games in my small town, many of my high school friendships faded quickly. Without the cozy confines of school it became so much more apparent that unless I was proactive, I'd spend the rest of my life going in a different direction than my peers.

I wanted to be more independent. I needed a plan—a place to go, people to see, work to do, a routine, a purpose, a van.

Because I didn't feel that I had much to offer, I didn't pursue any relationships with women. They were all nice, but going out on a date with me was a different story.

What was I going to do? Wheel up to some girl and introduce myself? "Hey, baby, I'm Duane. I live with my parents. I don't have a job or a car. In fact, I can't even drive, but my mom takes me everywhere I need to go. She also helps me when I need to go to the bathroom. So, how 'bout we go to the movies, you and me? My mom said she can take us either Friday night or Saturday. Whaddaya say?"

Why even ask? Why get my hopes up only to hear some line about what a great friend I am? That's me, good ole Duane. Everybody's friend.

A few people proposed that I try to meet a girl with SMA or MD. Anyone who suggests that to someone with a muscular disease hasn't really thought things through. What are we going to do, sit in the same room together and not be able to touch each other or take care of each other? Then you'd have two people in the same house who need to be cared for. I suppose if one of us were somehow wealthy and could pay a hundred grand a year for around-the-clock care for two people, it might be an option. It didn't make much sense to go out of my way to seek companionship with people like me. The MDA camps I went to as a kid were about the only times I did that. Gather more than one of us in any place for any length of time and you also need to gather more caregivers.

I realized the key to breaking out of the funk and getting the things I wanted was to get a job. I learned that if I had a job, I'd qualify for a government-subsidized grant to customize a van. I really wanted to go to work.

I knew my physical constraints and mobility issues would be concerns of any employer. In fact, I could think of only a handful of jobs that I could perform. So, instead of focusing on the things I couldn't do, I thought in terms of things I could do. I could think, speak well, talk on the phone, write, and move around most offices in a wheelchair. Computer terminals and PCs were starting to hit the workplace. I was capable of using computers.

I figured that working in an office would be only slightly more physically demanding than a day at school. But most jobs that I was able to physically perform required high levels of training or education. I had to work in an office that could accommodate my wheelchair. But I didn't have any experience. I needed someone to give me a chance—someone to show a little faith in me.

My First Job

"My van, my house, my wife, my son, my place in the community...my job made everything possible."
--Duane

Duane

I was rolling around at the Lindale Countryfest in October of 1984 when I struck up a conversation with the former County Sheriff, J.B. Smith. We knew each other as acquaintances but had never before had a substantial conversation. It wasn't long before the topic turned to work, more specifically my difficulty in finding a place that would give me a chance. I could tell from the tone of the conversation that we had moved beyond the point of idle chitchat.

J.B. Smith seemed genuinely interested in helping me network with people who might be able to help me. "Where all have you applied, Duane? What kind of work do you want to do?"

"I'm kinda focused on working close to home because I'd either have to roll to work in my chair or work out rides around my mother's job. I don't know how many places are able to work around my wheelchair."

"You seem to be a quick thinker, Duane. Does being an emergency dispatcher interest you?" J.B. asked.

My heart jumped with excitement just hearing the question. "You wanna know something funny Mr. Smith? I always wanted to be a cop. I suppose dispatching is about as close as I could get to that."

J.B. nodded in agreement. "Let me tell you a little story. The best dispatcher I've ever known, Mike Snider, is in a wheelchair. He once told me that he thinks being disabled actually helps him in his job. He said he's been in distress so often that it helps him relate well to people in desperate circumstances."

I knew exactly what Mike was talking about. I always thought I had good eyes and ears for people who need help. My problem was that I was rarely able to render help. As a dispatcher, all I would have to do would be to coordinate help. "Mr. Smith, I think being a dispatcher would be the perfect job for me."

"Tell you what, Duane, if I get re-elected come see me. We'll see what we can do."

To hear J.B. Smith rave about a disabled dispatcher was a thrill. To hear someone with hiring authority not be dismissive of my handicap was uplifting. To learn that someone like me had already proven himself in law enforcement planted the seeds of a master plan in my mind. I didn't know why I'd never thought about that work before. If I could get that kind of job, I could make new friends, save money for a van and qualify for a government grant for the working handicapped that would cover the cost of the van customization. Maybe I would even be able to save for my own house. And, with a job, money, and a van, maybe one day I'd actually take a girl on a date without my mom driving us around.

Three months later, shortly after J.B. Smith was reelected, an off-duty Smith County Sheriff's deputy dropped off a job application at my house. But by then I was already being considered for a dispatcher position at the Lindale Police Department. I knew Lindale well—the layout of the town and the people who lived there. The police department was less than a mile from my house so I could roll to work if I needed to.

In January of 1985, I was hired as a part-time dispatcher for police, fire, and ambulance services in Lindale. The police chief and city manager made a few minor accommodations in my workspace and I settled in quickly. For seven months I worked only on Thursday evenings and as a substitute for the full-time dispatchers. I was only making $4.20 an hour but for the first time in my life I was earning my own money. For the first time since high school, I felt like I fit in.

I started saving every penny of every paycheck for a van. After a few months, my parents chipped in and I picked out a new, shin, metallic-blue van with upgraded chrome wheels. But I was still a long way from driving. It took six months for the Texas Rehabilitation Commission, a government funded service, to process and approve my application for the adaptability grant. Meanwhile, when I worked third shift, my mom stayed up until midnight so she could drive me to my office. And, she was there in the morning to pick me up and take me home before going to her own job.

Finally, after all the paperwork was completed and installation of the lift and accessible driving controls were installed, we went to pick the van up. After getting a demonstration, I deployed the lift, loaded myself into the van, locked my wheelchair behind the steering wheel and operated a motor vehicle, without using a broomstick, for the first time. I can't imagine anyone ever being more thrilled than I was just to drive around the block.

I went to the DMV the next morning. With only the previous day's drive around the block and extensive video game experience, I was able to pass the test and get my license.

My van not only liberated me but also did the same for my mother. Once she got me dressed and out of bed in the morning, I was self-sufficient. A whole new world opened up to me. If I wanted to go somewhere or do something, I **told** my parents instead of **asking** them to take me. Six years prior, my first electric wheelchair gave me independent mobility within a limited range. My van took my independence to a new level. Once someone got me dressed and into my chair, I could go everywhere I wanted by myself without imposing on anyone. I still lived with my parents, but at twenty, I finally felt like an adult.

On August 4, 1985, I was hired fulltime as an emergency dispatcher for the City of Lindale. In addition to earning a living and the social benefits, the job forced me to exercise my muscles. Even though I was in a wheelchair, I had to type, answer phones, write, and perform general tasks around the office. Even sitting erect in my chair and talking is exercise to someone with SMA. Because of work, I dressed and drove five days a week. While working, I was more likely to go to the grocery store, run errands, and remain a part of the community.

My mobility was not only a morale boost but was therapeutic in my battle to hold the line against my disease for almost twenty years.

As the junior dispatcher on staff, I worked the least desirable shifts but I didn't care. I was independent. I didn't care too much about the low pay. Instead of being a tax burden, I was a taxpayer.

When a little girl went missing, I was the one who heard her father's panic. When someone walked into their home and found their mother, father, son, or daughter not breathing or without a pulse, I took the call and coached them through the worst moments of their lives. When a little boy called for help because his house was burning and he didn't know his address, I had to figure out where to send the fire trucks. When a battered woman called for help, she heard my voice first. When lives hung in the balance someone would dial 911 and ask me—a man who could barely move—for help.

I did everything I could to serve the people of Lindale in their darkest hours. Sometimes, there were happy endings. Sometimes the help they needed was beyond my means to provide. There were times I was powerless which, like my disease was a hard thing to accept.

Over the course of almost twenty years, I would talk to thousands of people in the most desperate and traumatic moments of their lives. Nothing connects a person to the human condition more than being a 911 dispatcher in a small town. From day one until my last day of work, I loved my job.

We've Fallen and We Can't Get Up

Duane

I answered the call like every other. "911, is your emergency police, fire or ambulance?"

The woman's voice on the other end carried a tone of distress. "Hello? We've fallen and we can't get up."

I'd taken many calls over the years from elderly women who have fallen down, but never from someone who has said "we've fallen."

As a dispatcher, the first things to clarify from the caller are whom and how severe. "Ma'am, how many people have fallen?"

Her voice trembled as she told the story. "My friend fell. Then I tried to help her up, but then I fell on top of her. She seems to be in pain. She says her hip hurts."

"Ma'am, I'm going to get you some help. What's your name?" The promise of help usually calms people instantly. So does personalizing the discussion.

"My name is Clara Johnson." The calming techniques seemed to have worked. She sounded like she was introducing herself over afternoon tea in the parlor.

"Okay, Clara. My name is Duane. Do you know the address where you are calling from?"

Within seconds of taking the call, I had an officer and an ambulance dispatched. I knew well the vulnerability and the anxiety that goes along with being on the ground with no strength to get up. Clara's predicament was one I had been in several times.

After graduating high school, I spent the weekdays by myself. My mom would get me up and put me in my wheelchair before she and my dad went to work and my sister went to school. In those days, my arms were strong enough that I could roll around the house, fix myself something to eat, go to the bathroom, even leave the house and roll around the neighborhood.

Although I had flipped my chair over several times and fallen out of it on a few other occasions, I'd never had any problems inside my own house. One morning, just after everyone had left, I was rolling from the living room toward the hallway when the right front toe plate of my chair rammed into the doorjamb. I went from two miles an hour to a dead stop instantly. My body went airborne. I tried to put my arms over my face but in addition to my arms being weak, they also move slower than other people's. My forehead hit the tile floor with a thump.

There I was, lying facedown like a turtle with no legs. Although my brace probably helped cushion the impact, it was causing a concentration of pressure on my chest. Instead of my weight being distributed across the whole front of my body, the full force of my body mass was pressing the hard, plastic brace into the hard, tile floor over a very small area of my chest. It wasn't long before my adrenaline drained and I realized I was having a hard time breathing. My body brace was squeezing the air out of my lungs like a boa constrictor. It was taking a lot of effort to breathe. I needed to get the pressure off my chest.

With my arms winged out beside me, I pressed my right forearm and elbow into the floor as hard as I could. That rolled me ever so slightly to the left, changing the pressure point by an inch or two. It brought momentary relief but it required tremendous exertion and as soon as I let up, I rolled back to the same point. I tried pressing my left elbow down to roll me the other way, but my left arm wasn't strong enough.

I couldn't see a clock, but it couldn't have been much past nine o'clock. It would have been a lot easier to breathe if I had been on my back, but I hadn't been able to roll over on my own since I was a child. I was expecting my mother home for lunch at about twelve. *Can I make it three hours?* I didn't know.

Maybe I can move. If I can move, maybe I could make it to a phone.

I pressed both forearms into the floor and tried to scoot forward. I could almost feel myself move. I tried again. This time I reached my chin out as far as I could and dug it into the floor and with all the might my neck could offer, drew my chin back toward my chest. I moved two inches!

My chin, nose, right cheek, left cheek, and forehead all took turns helping my elbows pull my body across the floor, like a slug in slow motion.

I bet it took me half an hour to make it into my bedroom. I saw my phone sitting on a bookshelf three feet above the floor so I made my way first toward a pool cue, which stood upright in the opposite corner of the room. I also saw the digital clock. It was 9:45.

I squirmed my way toward the stick and when I reached it, I laid it down in front of me. Then, I headed to the phone. In between pulling myself, I also pushed the pool cue along the floor, two inches at a time. By 10:15, I had moved across my room to the bookshelf. With both hands extended in front of me, I gripped the heavy end of the pool cue like I was holding a baseball bat. Then I swung the stick blindly above the back of my head. Framed pictures and books fell from the shelf and came bouncing down around me. Then I heard the "ding" of the rotary phone as it landed in my blindspot somewhere in the opposite direction that I was facing. *I'm sure glad that didn't land on my head.*

I lifted my head and turned it the other way. The phone was within reach, which meant so was my mother who worked only one mile away.

Within five minutes she was lifting me off of the floor. She put some kind of ointment on the abrasions on my elbows, chin, and cheeks and an icepack on my purpling eye.

I had a pretty good idea of how it feels to have fallen and not get up.

"Clara, would you like me to stay on the line with you until help arrives?"

"Oh, yes I would. Thank you, Duane."

"How long have you been on the floor, Clara?"

"I don't know. It took a long time for me to get to the phone."

"You want to know something funny, Clara?"

"What's that?"

"I've been in a wheelchair since I was twelve. I was in the same situation you're in now. I was on the ground for over an hour and used a pool stick to knock the phone down to me."

"Oh, bless your heart. We don't have a swimming pool."

I stayed on the line with Clara for a bit longer until I got word that our officer was arriving at the scene. "Clara, officer David Abbot is pulling into your driveway right now. Is your front door locked?"

She talked to her friend, then to me. "Tell him there's a key under one of the flower pots."

"Okay, I'll tell him."

"I hear his car." Her voice quivered as she repeated herself. "I hear his car, Duane!"

"You're in good hands, Clara. Officer Abbot will take care of you two. He will be entering your front door in just a few seconds."

"Oh, thank God. Thank you, Duane."

"Yes ma'am. Anytime."

A few days later, an old lady came into the police station. She had a big plate of chocolate chip cookies. I looked through the service window as she approached.

The lady who held the cookies saw me. "You must be Duane."

I recognized her voice. "You must be Clara."

People like Clara reminded me of why I loved my job.

Meeting Kim

Duane

I stopped for gas at my usual spot. I lowered my lift and rolled inside to get a cold drink. There was a new girl working the counter. I couldn't suppress my smile. "Hello"

She flashed a bigger-than-just-polite smile back. "Hi."

But I'm used to that. Strangers are almost always courteous to folks in wheelchairs. Everywhere I go, people smile and say "hi." Strangers sometimes act like they know me, so I'm often left wondering, "Do I know them?"

In the case of Kim, I knew I'd never seen her before. If I had, I would've remembered her deep blue eyes and long dark hair, but most of all, I wouldn't have forgotten her smile. Lindale was a small town and I knew she couldn't have been in town long or I would've already known who she was.

I wheeled back toward the cold drinks and pulled a soda off the rack. I rolled up to the counter to pay. I had to know more about her.

"Are you new to Lindale?"

"Yeah." She smiled again. "I moved from Waco a few months ago. My name is Kim."

"Nice to meet you, Kim. I'm Duane."

I couldn't get her out of my head so I went back the next night and bought another Coke.

After ten Cokes, I finally got the courage to ask her out. We both worked the evening shift so our first date started at midnight. Nothing was open so we just drove around town, talked, listened to the radio, and played *guess the song.* We were having a good time, but there was still a bit of uneasiness in not knowing each other very well.

Kim still lived with her parents and had a two o'clock curfew. I was driving her home when the DJ reminded us to set our clocks back an hour for the end of daylight savings time. Then he played a song. After only three chords, we both shouted in unison:

"If I Could Turn Back Time!"

"Jinx. You owe me a Coke." I said, instinctively.

We were both laughing so hard that Kim had a hard time speaking her response. "Owe you a Coke? I've already sold you ten of 'em."

The unexpected extra hour, the song, guessing at the same time, the Coke joke. We giggled like teenagers.

The moment was a real icebreaker. It turned the evening from *special* to *epic*. I turned the van around and extended her tour of Lindale by an hour. It was during that bonus hour when we became completely relaxed with each other. The conversation was so effortless. On our first date, I felt a chemistry that I'd never felt before. It's funny; my whole life I've felt like time was running out, but on that night it felt like time stood still. I guess it did, for one hour.

I called Kim the next day and most days after that. We talked a lot on the phone, but our work schedules kept me from asking her out again right away. Besides, I was pretty nervous about asking. One drive-around-town night was not that big of a deal, but I didn't want to risk being rejected for a second date.

Another thing concerned me. During our many hours of phone conversations, Kim still hadn't asked me why I was in a wheelchair. *Had she already been told by someone else? Did she know that my condition was a degenerative one?*

One night I stopped at the town pool hall and ran into a girl that Kim worked with at the store.

"Have you seen Kim tonight?" I asked.

"Yeah…didn't you know it was her birthday?" She replied.

"Oh yeah...I guess she mentioned it. Do you know where she is? I called her house but nobody answers."

"She went to the movies, by herself. She told me she hinted for you to take her."

I had blown it by not acknowledging her birthday, but at least now I knew she was interested in me. If she was going to the movies by herself on her birthday, clearly she was single. I went and bought a Coke the next day and asked her out again. From then on, we didn't let our work schedules get in the way of seeing each other.

In December, two months after our first date, I gave Kim a gold necklace, which led to our first kiss. We dated for four years while Kim earned an accounting degree in Tyler. Meanwhile, I continued to live at home and work at the police department.

In 1996, after six years of dating, Kim had shown she was in it for the long haul. In addition to being my girlfriend, she had already taken the baton from my mother as my primary caregiver.

I'd been saving for a ring for a while. I couldn't get down onto one knee but I wanted to propose in some unique way, so I asked Kim to put me in the recliner. I didn't want to propose from a wheelchair. I wanted us both to remember the uniqueness of the moment. I asked her to bring a sack to me. She had no idea what was inside. I asked her to kneel beside me so I could be at eye-level with her.

I was thrilled to see her excitement and elated when she said "yes". We had been together for six years. By this time, she knew what life with me would be like. She knew it would inevitably get harder on her. She knew all the work and care that went along with being my wife, yet she still reacted to the proposal like I was a prize.

Kim and I were married in September of 1996. I sat at the alter, surrounded by beautiful flowers, candles, family, friends, and coworkers in their police uniforms, but when I kissed my bride I felt as though we were the only ones in the church.

Kim was joy-crying. Seeing that reaction in her and a bigger version of that same smile on her face that I saw the night that I met her in the store was one of the happiest moments of my life.

I didn't endear myself to the bridesmaids when I rolled over Kim's dress on purpose, but what were they gonna do? Hit me?

Before I ever met her, if I were asked to conjure a prototype of the woman I needed, I would have come up with Kim—patient, pretty, mature, understanding, giving, tender, smart, and strong-willed. I needed to find someone who valued love over everything else put together and God put a very limited number of women like that on earth. Lucky for me, one landed in my little world of Lindale.

Holding Logan

"Logan is a gift from God. He is my world, my future, my legacy"
--Duane

Two months after Duane's wedding, his old friend, Ronald Bunch, took his family on vacation, and asked Duane to look after his house while he was gone. "Just keep an eye on it for me, Duane, would ya?"

"No problem, Ron. I'll collect your mail as well."

Twenty-four hours later, Duane was at work when a 911 call came in. "Is this Duane?"

"Yes sir, what is your emergency?" Duane asked.

"Duane, your buddy, Ron…his house is on fire!"

Duane dispatched the fire engines to his friends house, but it was too late. The house was a total loss, except the kitchen sink, which Ron's wife had installed in the their new home about the same time that Duane purchased the lot from the his old friend for one dollar. Duane had the house rebuilt on that property then he and Kim moved out of their apartment and into their own house the following spring.

Duane wants to let all readers know that if they would like to hire him to do a little house sitting, just let him know. He has references.

***

Having settled into their new lives, Kim started researching the possibility of them having a child. When they learned the odds were very slim that they'd have a child with SMA, they decided to try to get pregnant.

On Christmas Eve of 1998, Kim came to Duane with a big smile. "Guess What? We're having a baby!"

Duane was in the birthing room when his son, Logan, was born. His mother-in-law put a pillow on his lap and placed the tiny baby on the pillow. Duane looked in joy and amazement at what he and Kim had. He held his newborn son tight.

Duane already had a job, a van, a home, a wife, and now he had a beautiful healthy son. He felt as normal as his baby boy.

When he drove Kim to the hospital, they left the house as a couple. Two days later, they returned home as a family. Duane's life would never be the same. Not only had a community come to rely on Duane, now a child was depending on him.

Duane napped every day with baby Logan on his chest. When Logan got too big for that, Duane pulled his left leg onto his right knee and dropped him on his lap and rolled him everywhere in his wheelchair. When Logan got to big for that, he put him on the footrests. When Logan got to big for that, he rode on the back of his chair. When Logan gets to big for that, He will drive his father in the van.

Good Times Van

"I used to be an excellent driver."
--Duane

Using his electric wheelchair and specially-equipped van, for twenty years Duane was able to get from his driveway to his dispatch desk in downtown Lindale without assistance. Getting from his bed to his his driveway hasn't been as easy. Since ninth grade, every morning that he left the bed someone (first his mother, then his wife) strapped him into his brace, dressed him, lifted him into his wheelchair, and usually opened the front door for him.

On those occasions when he had to open the front door himself, he had to rely on his weaker arm to exit his house and enter the outside world. Duane's dance with the front door of his house was a choreographed routine. The ritual was made possible when his father installed a door lever, instead of doorknob, on the inside of his front door.

Like so many adaptations, his mind had to invent a clever way for his debilitated body to move a clumsy inanimate object (the door) without his own body or his wheelchair getting in the way. Duane's disease forced him to practice the basic principles of physical science. When you have less than a small fraction of the muscle strength of the average person, you come to understand the application of levers, torque, momentum, fulcrums, kinetic energy, and friction.

In his twenties, he could joystick his wheelchair forward and back to park along the inside of his front door. It took all his strength, but he was able to pull down on the well-lubed door lever with his left hand while bumping *reverse* with the joystick in his right hand.

Sometimes it took three or four attempts but eventually he'd pull the door off the latch so he could then use the left footrest of his wheelchair to draw the door fully open. He looked through the doorway at the rest of the world—the world outside the comfort of his walls—that despite not being adapted to suit his limitations was nonetheless a world he wanted to be a part of. Rolling through that doorway to access that world presented an immediate challenge: closing his front door.

As he slowly rolled his wheelchair past the open front door, with his left hand, he grabbed the nylon rope that was tied around the front-side doorknob. About four feet of rope slid through his hand as he eased forward until he felt the knot near the end of the rope. He made a tight, left fist around the rope, cut a hard right with his chair so he would roll on the concrete alongside his house instead of flying off the front porch into his equivalent of the Grand Canyon. At the mark, he'd let loose of the rope at about the same time the door slammed behind him. The hardest part of his day was over.

Getting into the van was easier than getting out of his house. He first pressed a button on his remote control that opened the rear, passenger-side door and lowered the lift. After wheeling his chair onto the platform and making sure the safety guides are raised, again using the remote, he raised the lift.

When the lift hit the home position, he rolled his wheelchair through the open space up to the spot in which the driver's captain chair used to be. The chair snapped and locked in a precise spot that enabled him to grip the custom knob on the steering wheel with his right hand and pinch the throttle and break lever between his left thumb and forefinger. He also had an electronic-touch gearshift and an easy-access key within reach of his right hand. Off he went, wherever he needed to go.

He felt comfortable with the routine and even though as years passed driving became increasingly challenging, most days went by without incident. Driving his own van meant independence and mobility, and it was something Duane could do for his son.

Duane's van connected him to the best times of his life: His job, his first date with Kim, and driving Logan to his activities. However, there were many times when things didn't go so well in the *Good Times Van*. When either his equipment failed or his hands lost their grips on the controls, the result ranged somewhere between a funny story and a close call with death.

One morning, Duane and Logan loaded into the van. Duane was planning to drop Logan off at school and then head to work. He shifted into reverse and started backing out of his carport. As the van rolled slowly backward down the grade of his driveway, his left arm bounced on its armrest and slipped backwards. It was only a one-inch shift, but was enough for his hand to slide off the brake lever.

The car was stuck in reverse and the man sitting behind the steering wheel couldn't move his hand forward even one-single inch to apply the brakes. Next to him sat a six-year-old child in a seat belt. The only control he had over the vehicle was his right hand's ability to steer it. So that's what he did. He fixated on his rear-view mirror and successfully swerved to avoid the tree trunk across the street from his driveway. The van picked up a little speed but he kept it on the road.

His mind scrambled for a solution as he tried with all his might to move forward in his chair just one inch. In avoiding the tree, he ran over two of the Quattlebaum's trashcans, wedging them between the rear bumper and the road. The scraping of the trashcans served as an auditory reminder of just how out of control the situation was as he narrowly missed running over Ronnie Davis's mailbox.

One hundred yards into his joyride and still rolling backwards at about two miles per hour, he saw three options in his rear view mirror. One of the following objects was eventually going to stop his van: The Harding's boat parked on the end of the street, the driver's side of Nathan Wilson's brand new white Ford F150 pickup, or the Jackson's chain-link fence. As most decisions do, it came down to money. He knew he didn't want to buy a truck or a boat, so he aimed for the fence.

Then he suddenly remembered about the passenger-side panic brake. "Hit that red button, Logan!" Duane pointed with his eyes to an emergency button that was part of the accessible package that he'd never used before and had forgotten about.

Ten feet before the van was going to run over a chain link fence, Logan unbuckled his seat belt and hit the red button. The van jerked to a stop. "Come push my arm up a bit Logan," Duane instructed his son.

Logan bent over him and shifted his father's forearm two inches forward so his hand gripped the lever.

With the help of his six-year-old son, Duane was able to drive him to school. "You want some donuts this morning, Logan?"

"Yeah!" Logan replied.

"Tell you what. If you promise not to tell your mom about this, we'll stop at the Donut Palace this morning."

***

Getting the van stuck in reverse at walking speed and buying new trashcans for the guy who mows your yard is a funny story. Having it stick in the full-throttle position could have been disastrous.

His van had gone from thirty to fifty before he realized what was happening. He didn't know that a plug in a control circuit had come loose, all he knew was that his throttle was stuck wide open and no amount of jiggling the lever was going to get it "unstuck."

Unless he did something, in about ten seconds he'd be screaming down the highway at eighty miles per hour. He let go of the steering wheel for a second and with his right hand flipped the parking brake switch. That created some drag but was no match for the 351 engine.

The brake held the car at fifty until it burned up and the smell of melted rubber filled the van.

He ran through a stop sign at high speed and was heading out of town. He looked down at his gas gauge. It showed half a tank. He and his van barreled down the highway. He started looking for a place to ditch the van. What he really needed was a Rocky Mountain style runaway truck ramp. *There has to be something I can do...*

Then it came to him. *Kill the engine.* “I don't know where I got the idea, maybe God spoke to me.” Duane said when recalling the story.

He turned the key one click counterclockwise. The engine died but the steering wheel continued to function and the van coasted maybe half a mile until it came to a rest mostly still on the narrow road. If the idea to turn off the key had not come to him when it did, he would have had a high-speed crash.

He loaded himself on the lift and lowered his chair onto the shoulderless road and drove his wheelchair one mile to his office. Relieved to be safe at work, he wheeled up to his dispatch desk. He was about to call the shop and tell them that the system they had installed in his van almost killed him when a 911 call came in. Some lady was complaining about her neighbor's barking dog. Duane responded in the usual manner. “I'll have an officer dispatched to handle your emergency.”

Close calls with his van became a way of life for Duane.

He was driving alone on a country road when he hit a pothole that was so big it shook him in his chair and he toppled over. From his right-leaning slump his eyes fell below the dashboard. He still had his right hand on the wheel and could turn it, but his left hand at gotten knocked off the throttle/brake. With his head below the dashboard, he couldn't see where he was going. When he rotated his head as far to the left as possible, he only saw three things: The car radio in front of his face, an expanse of blue sky through the windshield, and the tops of trees flanking each side of the blue sky. When he sensed the right side of his vehicle pattering on ground instead of pavement, he eased the steering wheel a little left.

It may sound like similar to the stuck-in-reverse scenario that began in his own driveway, but this crisis had many more elements of danger.

First, he couldn't see where he was going or what might be coming toward him from the other direction. Second, he was on a lonely, country road rather than in his neighborhood.

Third, nobody was with him, nor did anyone know where he was.

Fourth, it was one hundred degrees outside.

With the brake impossibly out of reach, Duane, from his cockeyed slouch, peered over the ridge of the dashboard and through the windshield and steered his van between the treetops as it slowed. But it was stuck in drive, so even if he could manage to keep it on the road for a bit it would keep going like the Energizer bunny.

He strained to reach the key with his right hand. He pinched the key between his thumb and forefinger and was able to kill the engine. The van coasted to a stop as the air conditioner kicked off. The van wouldn't crank when he turned the key.

He didn't know whether he was on the left side of the road or the right. All he could see was the center console of the van. He hoped he was straddling the yellow lines in the middle of the road because he figured that would increase the likelihood that someone would stop to see why a van is parked in the middle of the road.

He felt the searing heat of the sun shining on the left side of his face. The inside of the van heated up instantly. He knew that he had only a matter of hours before he'd start dehydrating and not long after that his brain would fry.

He didn't know if the next car to approach would stop and the driver render aid or whether hundreds of cars would pass before some curious motorist walked up to the van days later to discover his baked and blistered body.

Sweat ran down both sides of his tilted head and formed a steady drip point from his chin. After ten minutes, he heard the first car approach. He heard it slow down and the tire's crunching against the road. Unable to reach the horn, he yelled for rescue.

The other car kept going.

Ten feet away, other human beings were unknowingly driving right past a man in danger for his life. He figured his only chance of surviving this one was if someone happened to stop to check on his van during the next three hours. He figured his chances of that happening were pretty slim.

He twisted his head to the right to see how big the pond of sweat was below him. That's when he saw the emergency radio that he had installed years ago on the floorboard and ignored since then. He had no idea if the frequencies on the radio were still actively used. Thank God it powered on.

He heard a man's voice come from the radio. Duane, a man who had dedicated his life to helping others when they called him in distress, this time was the one asking for help. "Sir, I'm in a desperate situation. I'm in a wheelchair and I'm stuck inside my van on the side of the road. I'm getting really hot. Can you please help me get a hold of someone for me?"

The man pulled over to a payphone and made a call that saved Duane's life. His cousin, who ironically happened to live just a few hundred yards up the street, arrived at his van just a few minutes later. He propped Duane up in his chair, gave him a bottle of water and sent him on his way. "Don't tell my mom," Duane asked his cousin.

***

One afternoon in March of 1989, he parked his van in his designated spot behind the police department. His lift requires a lot of extra room, nearly the equivalent of two parking spaces.

He pushed the button to open the side door. He tapped the joystick on his wheelchair to position himself on the lift platform. The lip on the edge of the platform popped up as usual. Everything looked normal. Unbeknownst to Duane, the lip had not locked in the vertical position. Instead of his chair tapping the lip and then stopping, which, under normal circumstances alerted Duane that he was positioned correctly, the two front wheels rolled over the edge of the lift. The whole chair, with his body in it, followed.

Duane's brain sent signals down his spinal cord to tell his arms to extend, his head to turn, and his core and neck muscles to contract and tighten. Those signals hit dead ends in his spinal cord because there were no motor neurons to transmit the commands. The messages never made it to his non-existent muscles.

Somewhere in a different part of Duane's brain, he experienced the panic of falling toward pavement—a flash of terror, the anticipation of pain, the fear of death. He was falling toward the surface of the paved parking lot in a body that was no more capable of protecting itself from the impact or the resulting trauma than a falling apple would be from preventing itself from bruising.

As his head raced toward the pavement, he knew whether he lived or died was going to be left to some combination of luck and God's will. His body hit with a thud. Then his neck whipped his head into the hard asphalt. He was still conscious as his one-hundred-and-fifty-pound electric wheelchair dog-piled on top of him, breaking the bone in his upper left leg. Duane heard it snap like a thick tree branch. He screamed in pain.

No one heard his cries for help. In a small, sparingly-used parking lot behind the Lindale police station, a mangled, twisted mass of man and machine lay motionless. Unable to move, even to pivot his head to visually inspect his body, he knew he had survived the fall. Duane explains why he knew his life was still in danger.

"I couldn't believe I was still conscious. Actually, I was surprised to still be alive after falling that far. I

figured my chair must have hit first and absorbed a lot of the energy before my head hit. I was lying in a parking lot, seriously injured, fading in and out of coherent thought and there was nobody around to help. I knew my leg was broken, but I couldn't see whether the bone was poking through my skin. I worried that I had a compound fracture and blood was gushing out of my leg. The way my face was facing downward, I could barely see anything around me. On top of everything else, my glasses were gone and I'm practically blind without them. About all I saw was the pavement, blurry trees, and a little sky. All I could feel was pain and panic."

Less than one hundred feet away, cars whooshed by on the highway but nobody could see or hear him. The road noise from cars and the hustle and bustle of people muffled his pleas for help. It was like an Alfred Hitchcock plot—the noise of people preventing would-be-rescuers from hearing him.

The whole left side of his head was numb. Through the numbness, he sensed a warm liquid forming under the side of his head. To make matters worse, his left eye noticed a puddle of blood less than an inch beneath it. Where was the blood coming from? His ear, his face, his forehead? He had no way of knowing. Everything was blurry. Was his mind playing tricks on him? Was his head really lying in a puddle of his own blood? He closed his left eye, and opened his right. No puddle. A minute later, he did the same thing. This time his right eye picked up the leading edge of the growing pool of blood.

Worried that he might lose the one mechanism he had to call attention to his predicament—his voice—he started saving his yells. He tried not to think about how vulnerable he was. Hungry dogs, raccoons, and the greatest threat—fire ants. Just a few years previous, he had answered an emergency call of a distressed husband whose handicapped wife had fallen in her yard next to a fire ant mound. The lady died after hundreds of fire ant bites. *Do ants like blood?* He didn't know, but he knew buzzards did. A scene from the movie, *Conan the Barbarian,* flashed in his mind: Buzzards swooping down on a still-alive-but-motionless body.

His mind tried to recall the cars he saw a few moments before when he pulled into the parking lot. It was about 1:00 p.m. and he wondered if anyone might be returning from lunch soon.

He watched in terror as the blurry, leading edge of the blood puddle crept further away from him. A puddle of his own blood—reaching for infinity. How far would it flow before it took him to heaven? He didn't know.

He felt as though he might pass out, but strained not to, knowing his voice might be vital to getting help. How long had it been? Twenty minutes? An hour? He didn't know. Hope faded and acceptance started to set in. *I survived this fall and now I'm gonna die in a parking lot right in the center of town, right next to the old funeral home building.*

He heard a car door slam, maybe from behind him. He sensed a presence. "Help!" he screamed with all his breath.

He heard a man's voice. "Oh my God!" Rapid footsteps approached. He still couldn't see the man.

• • •

When he stood next to Duane, the man's feet were level with Duane's eyes. The man bent over and his face appeared. "Are you okay? What can I do?"

"Get this wheelchair off me." Duane said.

The man lifted the wheelchair off Duane and hurried inside to the police department. Duane's coworkers came rushing out to attend to him. They did what he normally does. "They called the ambulance."

The paramedics, whom Duane had sent on hundreds of calls over the years, arrived on the scene a minute later.

Duane couldn't see or touch any of his injuries. The only mechanism he had to judge their severity was pain. He asked his paramedic friends for information. "How does my leg look? Is it broken?"

"It's pretty swollen, so I'm going to cut your sock off so I can check your pulse in your lower leg."

"How does my head look?" He asked.

"Well...I think your nose is broken."

Duane asked the paramedics to alert his parents.

"They put his neck in a brace, strapped him onto a hard, wooden backboard, and rushed him to Mother Frances Hospital.

His mother and father were already there when Duane was pulled from the ambulance at the hospital. Their presence gave him comfort. By the time his boss, Police Chief Ron Carroll, arrived a little later, Duane was in stable condition and the staff was working on his broken leg. "I don't think I'm gonna be able to make it to work today," Duane said to his boss with a grin.

"Don't worry about it Duane, I'll put you down for one sick day. But tomorrow…no excuses."

Three months later, Duane drove himself back to work, clocked in and resumed his role as the voice of rescue in Lindale.

Two Rings

To many, their job is a paycheck. To Duane it was so much more. His job gave him a sense of value and service and was his social connection to the community. Besides the income and the psychological and social benefits, the physical grind of work slowed the decay of his muscles. As the years rolled by, getting out of bed, getting dressed, driving himself to work, feeding himself, all little tasks that most of us perceive as sedentary, became vigorous activities to Duane.

As his body weakened, things that were once easy got harder. He started to worry about the safety of the community. It wasn't often but when there were big wrecks, fires, or bad weather, phones rang off the hook. Sometimes all the incoming 911 lines would ring simultaneously. As Duane neared forty, he knew he had to make the decision on when to give up his job.

Answering all the calls was not a problem, picking up all the phones quickly was. Every caller thinks they are the only one reporting. Speed and physical agility are needed. During high call volume situations, Duane was not as fast as a healthy person would be. By this point he only had one useable hand. Once it took him almost a minute to answer the fifth phone call reporting the same traffic accident. The voice on the other side was impatient. "Geez, are you sleeping up there or what?" The caller asked. Duane had always prided himself on answering within two rings. That's when he started seriously self-assessing his nimbleness on the job. He reached a point at which he couldn't deny it any longer.

At forty, he had to confront perhaps the biggest *last* of his life—his last day at the police department. After a twenty-year battle, SMA had finally taken away his job.

There were a lot of other *last times* that went along with his last day on the job: The last time he earned a paycheck, the last time he was asked his professional opinion, the last time he would run an errand while he was on his way home from work, the last time he would ever answer a phone to hear a distressed voice on the other end of the line say, "Duane, I need your help!"

***

His friends held a retirement party at the community center. There were pictures and decorations, a moneytree that friends and coworkers filled with lots of cash, and there were speeches. No speech was more memorable than the one given by one of his closest friend's on the police force, Officer David Craft.

The lives of David Craft and Duane Hale intersected at many points. In 1989, when Duane was lying crumpled and broken-boned in the parking lot of the police station, David Craft was in the small group who came rushing out the the police station to aid Duane. It was Craft who calmed Duane the most.

Five years later, Officer Craft was working the wet and rainy scene of an accident. While seated in his patrol car, on the shoulder of Interstate 20, another vehicle, traveling at typical interstate speed, slid out of control and smashed through the rear of his police car. When both vehicles came to a screeching halt, Officer Craft lie fully conscious in the front seat, showered in glass, the rear bumper of his car resting in the back seat, his L-5 vertebra broken, and his police radio right beside him.

He clicked the radio and called his friend. "Duane, I've been in an accident. Send an ambulance."

X-rays revealed not only a broken back but also a tumor on his spine. The broken disc was the least of his problems. The specialist who consulted with him about the tumor removal was frank. "Unless we remove the tumor, you will die. When we remove the tumor, there is a strong possibility that you will either be paralyzed below the waist or on your left side. It's highly unlikely you will ever be able to return to the police force."

After nine months, Duane's buddy came back to the police force not only to serve Lindale but to grease Duane's little office ramp with WD-40 so his wheels would spinout, and to crawl up behind his wheelchair and disconnect a battery lead as Duane sat unknowing at his desk. For another ten years, the two would enjoy playing pranks and jokes on each other.

David Craft started his keynote speech at his friend's retirement party. "When I was told I might not walk again, I looked to Duane for inspiration. I thought about all the things he does without walking."

David paused and sniffled. "I even thought to myself, 'if I'm going to be in a wheelchair, I want to have an attitude like Duane's.' I resolved that if I was blessed to walk again, I would never take my health for granted. It's been over ten years since I came back to work after my accident and seeing Duane every day at the office has reminded me of my resolution."

David gave up his struggle to hold back tears as he ended his speech by speaking to his good friend and favorite coworker directly. "Duane, for all the times that you've sat in your chair, including right now, and you think you're looking up at me…you should know something. I'm looking up to you."

***

Beginning the day after Duane retired, most of the time he had spent in his wheelchair was replaced with time in his bed.

He went from working closely with a group of friends and talking to twenty different people every day to sitting in bed all day with nobody around. With Duane's wife at work and his son in school, Duane found himself at home all day, and just like his post-high-school year, looking for a sense of purpose.

At least this time he had his wife and son and was in his own home. At least at forty he could reflect on successes and accomplishments. He could look at his family, his home and his community and think, "Look what I've done." At least he had secured a place in the world.

Duane still had a few friends that got him out. Jerry and Hope Gaskill have four biological children, five adopted kids, and raise foster children. They frequently include Duane and Logan in their Brangelina-type family outings. Duane and Jerry have spent many evenings fishing the night away on the Gaskill's barge on Caddo Lake.

For two years after retiring from the police department, the biggest event of his day was when he got to do what only a few other dads did—pick his son up from school. That may not sound like a big deal, and to most people it's not a big event as much as it is a chore.

For him to pick his son up meant Kim had to take a late lunch. Not only did she come home during her lunchbreak to feed herself and Duane but she also got her husband dressed, into his chair, out of the front door, and saw him safely into his van. Then she'd head back to her office.

As Kim drove her car back to work, Duane would drive his van around town for nearly an hour until it was time to pick up Logan. That's a lot of trouble for a couple to go through when there are easier ways to get Logan home, but it was a big deal to Duane. Kim understood this, which is why she put forth so much effort to facilitate it.

Duane knew that he was in his last days of driving. He was running over trashcans and despite his best efforts his turns were getting sloppy. He wanted to milk every possible after-school-pickup out of his body before he gave up the keys forever. To be there when his son came running out of the building and jumped into the van with a smile on his face, showing off a finger painting of dinosaurs, or a telling him about the 100 that he made on a spelling test were memories he wanted before he would concede driving his van to SMA. Finally, Kim told Duane that she was tired of buying everyone in town new trashcans. Duane got in his van and picked Logan up after school for perhaps his most difficult *last time* to accept—his last time to drive.

Since retirement, when he awakes, he tries to think of a reason to get out of bed. It requires more effort now. His body melts so comfortably into the bed. The sheets caress his body. To lie in bed is easy and no one would blame him for doing so all day long. No one would think he's lazy or would judge him for doing nothing—for being nothing. He has a get-out-of-jail-free card…no…a stay-in-bed-free card. Every day he looks for a reason to not play that card. Today, he has plenty of reasons. He is writing, marketing, networking, and scheduling. He's placing and promoting *Life Rolls On* merchandise. Duane is not only raising awareness of his disease in a very personal and informative way by coauthoring this book, but in doing so, he is earning money again, helping to support his family again and saving for his son's college.

As a result of the notoriety brought about by this book release announcement, he has received a job offer that he will consider after the book is published.

The pre-launch publicity has already resulted in emails and Facebook friend requests from parents of SMA children seeking his advice and experience. If fighting SMA were a martial art, Duane would be a black belt of the highest degree.

***

The day before Duane's forty-sixth birthday, Duane's mother joined us to help us write about his childhood visits to an endless stream of doctors. While every birthday is a not only a milestone but also a gift for Duane, each one brings his parents closer to a reality that at one time seemed incomprehensible. As Peggy finished relating the story of Duane's childhood prognosis, she glanced at her son whose once blonde hair had turned gray. "After his father and I heard those doctors' predictions when he was little, I never imagined that forty years later we'd be worried about how Duane would manage if he outlived us."

His parents invited him and his family over for a birthday dinner. He could easily decline and say he doesn't feel up to it or turn the invitation around and ask them to come to his place, but he wants to show his father that he's doing just fine and he wants to get out of the house. So he goes.

During the process of immersing myself in Duane's life for three months, I couldn't help but wonder about the answers to the same questions his parents ask themselves. Will Kim and Logan be able to handle him as he becomes even more dependent and his mother ages? What if something happens to Kim? Logan dreams of going off to Texas A&M and becoming a vet. He's a smart boy and does well in school. If he stays on track, he may go off to college. How will Duane handle his son leaving home?

One day there will be no more of Logan's baseball games or band performances to attend. What will get Duane out of his bed then? How long is it before he can no longer be left alone?

From his bed, he can still move his head and right arm to shoo a fly, drink, use the phone and computer.

Like so many things that Duane used to be able to do, those things will join the list of things he can no longer do. How will he manage without his main connection to his world—his computer?

While his friends and family may wonder and worry about the uncertainties in his future, Duane has lived his whole life overcoming them.

Imagine You Are Duane

"I don't fit in a baby bath."
--Duane

When healthy people see a disabled man such as Duane, we probably think about some things he can't do, and it saddens us because we consider what those limitations would mean to us. Recreational pursuits likely come to mind first. He can't play sports, walk in the garden, or decide to take up new hobbies like painting or woodworking or revisit ones he used to enjoy such as photography and playing music. "Man, I bet he never has any fun," we think to ourselves.

A few of us might take a moment to ponder how he handles functional things like eating, going to the bathroom, intimacy, or his inability to access a world built for people like us. That's about as much thought most of us give before we resume shopping, eating, texting, working, or whatever it is we were engaged in before we encountered Duane.

Imagine for a moment what it's like to be Duane. If you get an itch on your ear, need a drink of water, or decide that you don't like your arm where it is, you have to ask someone else to help you.

If you wake up during the night and feel the need to go to the bathroom or to simply adjust your sleeping position, you have to wake up your partner and ask them to help you. Suppose you just got in an argument with your partner. The last thing you want to do is ask for help. But you have no choice

SMA progressively takes its victim's ability to cough. This means that if Duane gets any kind of virus, cold, flu, or infection, he is unable to clear his own breathing passages. For someone who can't cough, a common cold can evolve into something much more serious. Sniffles and colds that other people might be able to cough away have put Duane in the hospital and threatened his life. Next time you get a bad cold, imagine getting through it without coughing.

Unless we've been close to someone in Duane's condition, we can't begin to fathom how vulnerable he is in the world that we take for granted. We don't think about his inability to defend himself against ever-present threats.

What if you were sitting outside, alone in your backyard and felt the sting of an ant bite? You shake your leg, swat the biting ant and his army of friends off our body and go about your business. But what if you couldn't move your arms or legs? What if your only hope of not being bitten to death by fire ants is to push a joystick with your finger and hope the relays and motors in your wheelchair don't fail and can take you to another human being who happens to be close enough to brush the ants off your body? Next time you find yourself being swarmed by a few ants, imagine you are completely unable to move.

Most of us don't live in constant fear of gravity. If we slip or trip, we simply use our arms as shock absorbers while our friends laugh at our clumsiness. When Duane falls or his chair tips, hitting his head is a certainty. It's only a matter of how hard. The next time you brace a fall with your arms imagine afterwards what would've happened if your arms had the compressive strength of wet noodles.

Even the act of getting out of bed is a risk to Duane's safety. Several times he and Kim have tumbled to the floor together. When they do, it's usually her body that takes the brunt of it.

In his own shower, he once slipped between a mounted chair and the tile wall. He was wedged so tight that Kim had to call his father to help her pry him out.

How many times in your life has a barking dog threatened you? To dogs, wheelchairs are like cars, only a lot slower and easier to catch. The next time a German Shepherd or any other big dog presents a threat to you, imagine the helpless feeling you'd have if you couldn't use your arms or legs to fend it off. You'd be completely at the mercy of an animal. Aggressive dogs present a huge threat to Duane. Imagine if every unleashed, barking dog you happen to encounter were a Grizzly Bear. That's what it's like to be Duane

Coaching Through the Window

I was working late one night at Duane's house. When I went out to my car I saw that I had a flat tire. Duane asked if we could coach Logan as he changed the tire. Logan did the whole thing, following Duane's instructions while Kim watched. I realized that just like everything else he did, Duane had to seize opportunities to father his son. Even though he couldn't lift a lug wrench, that flat tire was a chance for him to teach his son.

While other kids had their dads lift them to the monkey bars, Duane used his chair as an extension of the playground by putting it under the bars and having Logan stand on it to reach them. When Duane was trying to teach Logan how to ride a bike, he intercepted him with his wheelchair before he wobbled out in front of a car.

Until Logan was in fourth grade, Duane would sit in his chair and watch Kim play catch with their son. Kim is quite an accountant but she didn't spend her childhood catching baseballs. By the time he was ten, Logan was throwing too fast for Kim. After one of his fastball's ricocheted off her glove and smacked her on the forehead, giving her two black eyes, the family decided to hire a local coach to give Logan private baseball lessons.

Duane had a lot of fun around town with Kim's swollen, purple face. At Brookshire's, some friends approached the couple while they were grocery shopping. "Oh my God, Kim! What happened to your face?" Even though the lady asked Kim, she seemed to look suspiciously at Duane for an explanation of why his wife had two black eyes.

"Hey, I didn't raise a hand to her." It was that kind of humor that puts people at ease around Duane. If he senses someone is awkward with his condition, he might make a joke about it.

He finds it easy to talk to children because there's rarely pretense and they tend to speak what's on their mind. Children are sometimes conduits to his making friends with their parents. Moms cringe and admonish their kids when their little ones let their curiosity get the best of them. One boy asked Duane at the grocery store, "Why are your legs so small?"

"Because I didn't eat my vegetables," Duane said.

The lady was embarrassed and apologized profusely. Within a few moments she was laughing with Duane. Meanwhile, her son gathered broccoli and carrots and threw them into the shopping cart.

Since his retirement, Duane spends a lot of time in bed, which he is strategically situated against a big window facing his front yard. Even on days that he never leaves the house, his bedroom window allows him a constant view of a small piece of the outside world. Duane had Logan's spring-loaded pitch back net set up just outside that bedroom window.

Passers-by might think they see a boy in the front yard, by himself, throwing a ball into a net contraption and catching the fly balls and grounders that it kicks back to him. They probably don't notice the boy's father, propped up in his bed with his head a couple of feet behind the open window, peering out, coaching his son, encouraging him as he hones his skills. "Keep your glove down on those grounders, Logan. Don't let it sneak under your glove. Keep the ball in front of you...Good, that's the way!"

Duane's main reason for getting out is to attend his son's activities, primarily baseball games. At the ballpark, Duane sits in his chair and watches other dads play catch with their sons, warming up their boys before the game begins.

He allows himself to close his eyes and enter a portal to his past—a window in time that has long since closed. His mind conjures up a memory he forgot he had.

There's a little boy with curly blond hair poking out from under a Texas Rangers ballcap. The images become vivid; the scene is detailed as his thoughts begin to take life and flow like a movie.

He's watching a nine-year-old version of himself—part embellished memory, part daydream. He's viewing the scene through someone else's eyes as he watches little Duane smile as he throws the ball to his dad. His mind integrates the real sound of a fastball striking a glove near him on the ballfield into a vision of the little Duane's throw slapping into his father's glove thirty-five years before.

He hears a real-time voice. "Nice throw, son. Put a little pepper on it."

But in his daydream, he processes that voice as his father's.

⚾ ⚾ ⚾

The ball zips toward the nine-year-old Duane and the vision becomes more surreal as his mind shifts the reverie to a new point-of-view. He's seeing things as little Duane. His dad's throw is hard but he's not afraid of it. He extends his left arm, flicks his glove and snags the ball out of the air. He hears the pop of the ball in his mitt and feels a slight sensation of heat on his palm.

One of the dad's at the ballpark yells. "Good catch, son".

But in his mind's eye, the voice of encouragement belongs to his father's.

He brings his gloved left arm across his chest to meet his right hand, grips the ball and jiggles it slightly and effortlessly so he's got two-fingers on the seams. He cocks his arm and slings it forward like Nolan Ryan. He feels the seams across his fingertips as the ball leaves his hand and watches it arc toward an outstretched glove. The ball hits the glove with a loud snap.

A kid's voice complains. "Not so fast, dad."

In his vision, the boy's voice is Logan's. He sees the respect for his fastball on his son's face.

The imagery seems so real. He's no longer playing catch with his dad; now he's playing catch with his son. The illusion begins to fade and a man's voice shakes him out of his trance and snaps him back to reality. "Logan, want me to warm you up?"

His son's voice is filled with enthusiasm. "Yeah, thanks Mr. Anderson."

Duane turns his head just in time to see his son catch a baseball and hear the distinctive thud indicating Logan caught the ball heavy on his palm instead of in the glove's webbing. Logan forces a smile as he objects to the fastball. "Ouch, not so fast, Mr. Anderson."

A Rare Kind of Kindness

On one of my visits to Duane's house, I brought lunch from *Simply Berties*. I took the food back to the place where most of the eating happens in the Hale home, around Duane's bed. I unloaded my wrapped meal and drink and placed it on the windowsill at the foot of his bed and put Logan's food on the edge of Duane's service tray, which is always butted up against his bed.

Duane was lying in his usual daytime position—a thirty-degree incline. He asked me to raise his bed higher to prepare for his meal, and then guided me on how to arrange his food. "Open that box and put it on my chest right here." He tapped his right forefinger on his upper sternum, just a few inches below his chin.

It seemed odd, to spread food out on a man's bare chest but I followed his instructions, setting the box-with-burger exactly where he asked.

"Now, put the straw in my drink and put it on the edge of the table so I can reach it."

Then he called for his son, who was in the living room. "Logan, your lunch is here."

Logan walked into the room. He smiled at me, respectfully. "Thanks for lunch," he said.

He made a beeline for a box of French fries on the bedside table. He grabbed a few and poked them into his father's mouth. He waited for Duane to chew and swallow and then fed him more. After about seven doses of fries, Logan grabbed his dad's drink and guided the straw toward his father's waiting lips. After Duane drank, he was able to grab the sandwich off his chest and take a bite.

Only after ensuring his father had eaten some French fries, had something to drink, and had a good grip on his sandwich, did Logan unwrap his own food.

Even after starting to eat, Logan continually put his burger down to stuff more fries into his father's mouth. Duane is not as fast an eater as most of us. It takes him twenty minutes to eat what we might eat in five, but Logan stayed in the room until his dad swallowed the last bite of his burger.

A little later in the afternoon, Logan came back into the bedroom and asked his father if he could go a block away to his friend's house.

"Go ahead." He looked at the empty, plastic urine bottle sitting in the windowsill as he smiled at me. "Don't worry, Rich'll take care of me if I needtah go pee."

I studied Duane to see if he was serious. He was smiling ear-to-ear.

"Uhm…maybe you should help your dad go pee before you leave," I suggested to Logan.

Just before he left, Logan popped back into the room. "I've got my phone with me." It was his way of reminding his father that even though he would be a block away, he was still available with a push of a button.

Growing up with the combination of a mother who demonstrates compassion every day and a father who can barely move has developed in Logan a level of empathy for the human condition that few children his age grasp.

I took the opportunity of Logan's absence to ask Duane about his son. Now that he's getting bigger and stronger, is he helping more with your care?"

Duane smiled. "Last night, when we went to Kilgore for Logan's game, it was the first time I've been out since Kim's surgery. Since she can't lift me right now, Logan operated the lift and got me out of my chair and into bed. It was the first time he's ever done it alone."

This was a huge milestone for the whole family. Having a second person in the house who is able to help Kim with the heavy lifting makes things a little easier on everyone.

***

"I am so proud of him," Duane said. "Back in third grade, his teacher told me that there was a girl in class who had some special needs. She had autism and a lot of other kids picked on her. She'd been having a hard time making friends. When Logan saw what was going on, he started sitting with her at lunch…"

During the middle of Duane's story, Kim came home for her lunch break. She instinctively grabbed the water cup next to Duane's bed—the one I hadn't noticed was empty—and refilled it. When she returned from the kitchen moments later, she stood next to her husband, appropriately enough, at his right hand.

She touched his shoulder tenderly and added to Duane's story in a way that I've noticed they both tend to do with each other when recalling events—a synchronized conversation that during these kind of discussions made it seem they were each speaking from a common brain. I could see how emotional Kim was as she joined the conversation. "The teacher said that she'd overheard him sticking up for the girl when other children talked cruel about her."

Kim tended to Duane, adjusting his legs to new spots. "She said she's seen him do that with more than one kid in class and that she'd hardly ever seen that kind of behavior out of third graders before. She said he has a rare kind of kindness."

"I can't imagine where he gets that from," I said to Kim with a sarcastic-complimentary smile.

"It made us feel like we were on the right track, you know?" Duane said, as he took his turn speaking.

"We aren't saying he's a perfectly behaved kid, because he's sure not." Kim said. "But he has something inside him that causes him to be protective and caring.

Logan had been gone about thirty minutes when Duane's phone rang. He can't hold the handset against his ear so he puts all his calls on speakerphone.

I heard Logan's voice coming over the phone. "Dad? I was just making sure you were alright."

"No! I'm stuck in my bed and I can't move!" Duane smiled at me as he teased his son.

"Dad…quit it."

"I'm okay, Logan. Thanks."

The Good in People

"Hey…you think you can loan me twenty bucks just 'til I can get back on my feet again?"
--Duane

Duane

My support network reaches beyond family. Perhaps partly as a function of being in a wheelchair, I am lucky to have collected a great number of friends.

After high school, one of my lifelong friends, Karen Dickerson, went off to college, then med school before setting up practice in Houston and Dallas. For more than twenty-five years, her trips back to Lindale often include a stop at my house. During one of her visits we were talking about a new aquatics facility that had opened in town. I was comparing the new mega pool to the one in which she and I had learned to swim. "Remember when you and Cassie would come over and play in our little four-foot, above-ground pool?"

"Oh yeah, I remember thinking that pool was so big," Karen replied. "Sometimes, when I see one of these pools now, I think of us. Duane, when was the last time you've been in a pool?"

"I don't know, Karen. It's been many years."

"Wouldn't you like to go to that pool at the aquatic center?"

"Sure I would, but they don't have a lift system."

"What do you mean, a lift system?"

"Well…they have these lifts for disabled people that lowers and raises them in and out of the pool…"

Karen contacted the manager of the facility and proposed to purchase and donate the lift to the aquatics center. In the end, they declined to accept her offer. I still haven't gone swimming since we spoke that day.

When she saw my legs were starting to draw tight, Karen had special braces delivered to stretch the ligaments and tendons in my legs. Kim put me in the braces for a short time each day. I built up my pain tolerance from one hour up to four but each prescribed session turned into a painful exercise in clock-watching. Progress was only incremental. After six months of intense no pain-no-gain therapy, I finally gave up. I felt like I had let Karen down more than myself. Karen's kind heart and my mother's experience working for other physicians who showed patience for the disruptions my care created during her workdays helped restore her faith in doctors.

I have to be careful when I talk to my old friend, Karen. If I insinuate that I'm lacking something, she might go out and buy it. *Karen, you know what would make my life so much better? A case of M&M's with Peanuts.*

• • •

Shortly after I got my first wheelchair, Billy Brewster's mother, Jimmie, saw my mother laying down a series of aluminum ramps next to our van outside Ferguson's Grocery Store. Jimmie shook her head as she watched my mom strain to push me up the ramp before loading our groceries. I sat in the van and heard Jimmie talking to my mom. "Oh, Peggy, they have automatic lifts for his chair, you know."

"I know Jimmie, we're saving up now. We'll need one pretty soon, he's getting so heavy."

Jimmie knew from experience the emotional and financial strain that my disease brought to our family. "Peggy, I know how much work it is to lay those ramps out by hand every time. And in the summer those ramps get so hot you can't even touch them."

Shortly after that downtown encounter and two years after her own son had passed away from MD, Jimmie solicited enough donations from citizens and small businesses around Lindale to buy us a wheelchair lift. We watched her husband, Donnis, install the same kind of lift in our van as he had for his son.

I'll never know who gave ten, twenty, or a hundred dollars to help our family when we needed it. In a way, I guess I kind of like it that way because I've always assumed it could be anybody I see.

It's not only family and close friends who look out for me. One of the few advantages of being in a wheelchair is that you tend to bring out the best in people. People go out of their way to hold doors for you. Strangers tend to be friendlier.

In 2008, I got a strange phone call. "Duane, my name is Phil Parham. I saw you and your son at the

Dollar Store on Saturday. I asked around town about you and your family."

This guy sounded too nice—like a salesman. I expected the next words to come out of his mouth were going to be something like, "Have I got a deal for you." What he said next caught me off guard.

"Duane, I called to ask you if there is any way I might help you. Is there anything hard about your life that I can make easier?"

"I'm not sure I understand what you're asking or offering Mr. Par—"

"Please call me 'Phil'. If you tell me what you need, I'll try to find the right charity or donors to get it for you. Is there something I can help you with? New wheelchair batteries, accessibility equipment, van repairs? Is there anything that you've been needing but don't see how you could afford it?"

"Okay, Phil, so you're not gonna try to sell me insurance or annuities?"

He laughed. "No. It is what I say it is: An offer to help you and your family. There are limitations to my offer so don't tell me you need a Corvette."

At first, I tried to tell Phil Parham that I was doing fine and that I needed nothing. But he was persistent. "There must be something you need, Duane. I feel like you're holding back on me."

There was actually something we had needed for some time—a lift system in my bedroom. My wife and mother's backs were under constant stress from lifting me in and out of bed. Sometimes I'd slide out of their grips and hit my butt on the floor during a failed attempt to transfer me between my bed and wheelchair or between my bed and my bathroom chair.

"Phil, you know there is one thing that would really help me and my wife…"

"I'll check on this for you, Duane."

The next day a man called to inspect and measure my room. Two days after that, a team was at my home installing a ten-foot rail on the ceiling from which hung a lift system, including all the webbing and straps we needed. A salesman from the company came out to demonstrate how to operate the system.

The whole process moved so fast, I wondered how Phil was able to secure the money and get it to come together so quickly. The websites I checked sold these types of lifts for several thousand dollars. I was more than curious about who paid for this so I tricked the salesman into telling me how it was paid for.

"Phil's wife, Peggy, already wrote a check," he said.

It seems there were no charities or groups of donors. For the stranger who saw me at the *Dollar Store* to imply otherwise was probably just a tactic to make me comfortable disclosing what I really needed. This seems to be a simple case of a man who reached out to another man whom he sensed was in need of something—something that, incidentally, one doesn't find at the *Dollar Store*.

When my van started overheating one hot summer day, I managed to pull into the parking lot of a gas station in Mineola, Texas, a town about fifteen miles away from home. I deployed my lift and was circling the van, contemplating how to get back to Lindale when a man I knew from my hometown pulled up next to me in his pickup truck.

Jack Roach was better known back in Lindale as *Cactus Jack.* He was renowned for his country demeanor, his roadside vegetable stand *Taters and Mators,* and his kind heart. "Duane, you look like a fella tryin' to git back to Lindale."

Jack grabbed an ole' boy from the parking lot and together they hoisted my chair into the bed of his truck and me into the cab.

When he dropped me off at work, I insisted he take ten bucks for his trouble.

Cactus Jack had a different idea. "Duane, next time you see somebody stranded, help 'em out. I'd rather you do that than give me money."

It wasn't long after, I heard from a local mechanic that there was a stranded man in a wheelchair at his garage. I didn't forget Cactus Jack's request. I drove to the shop and lifted the man and his chair into my van. As we passed the Mineola gas station on our to his house in Quitman, I told him the story of my own breakdown. Before I deployed the lift and lowered him to his driveway, he offered to pay me.

"Nope. Remember my story? I'll just ask you the same thing Cactus Jack asked of me. Just help out the next guy."

Pulling, Pushing, Tugging and Lifting

"In the advanced stages of our diseases, we can require more effort to care for than an infant. We might not cry for our caregiver's attention, instead we yell their names across the house from our beds.
--Duane

If there's one thing that I'll take away from working on this project above all else, it's the respect I gained for the caregivers. Whether family or professional, providing care for someone who can't move is not only a physically demanding and time-consuming job, but also requires learned skills.

The attitude of the caregiver and the quality and effectiveness of the care is a major factor in maintaining the spirits of their patients. MD, SMA, ALS, and these muscle diseases are not rehabilitation situations in which the patient makes progress and works toward a goal of getting better. These conditions are degenerative and incurable, and both the caregiver and the patient know the need for care will continue to increase until end-of-life.

Besides his own determination and resolve there's another reason that a man who can't move is usually seen with a smile and known for his positive attitude and good humor. It's the level of care he has received in his life, first, primarily from his mother, and then from Kim. If ever during my life, I need constant care, I could only hope to receive the kind that Duane has.

Whether dressing, moving, lifting, feeding, or cleaning, everything is done in a certain way. One needs to know where to pull, push, tug, and lift, and in what sequence. On several occasions, an inexperienced helper has dropped Duane's arm or leg after lifting it. "After they raise or lift my arm or leg, it's funny how many people let go. They don't realize I can't lower my arms or legs anymore than I can raise them. So gravity kicks in and I pop my elbow on a dresser or my foot onto something hard."

Duane knows the best way to do everything regarding his care. Even though he has never done it himself, he taught Kim. As his body has weakened over years, their techniques have evolved. The two have figured out new methods and have adapted, one might say as a "team". If anyone other than Kim helps, they might hear a series of commands. "Stand here, place your shoulder against mine, reach around the back, not the front, lift harder, use your other hand for that, do not let go of my arm until I say…"

Shortly after Duane and I started collaborating on this project, I began going to his home to work with him. It took my being at his bedside for several days before I fully understood just how much care he requires and the amount of devotion his wife has. On the rare occasions in which something keeps Kim from tending to one of Duane's needs, his mother is always just a few minutes away. While Kim takes care of Duane, most nights Peggy takes care of dinner. Sometimes she brings cooked meals over from her house. Other times she comes over to her son's kitchen and cooks for two households.

One might think that when Duane is at home, his wife lifts him easily out of his wheelchair to relax in a more comfortable recliner. She doesn't. Because of the extra exertion which would be required and because other chairs and couches just aren't really built to provide the assisting support Duane's body needs, he is always in one of three places: His bed, his wheelchair, or his bathroom chair.

Duane is heavy. Moving him takes a great deal of strength, force and leverage. Want to know what it's like to move Duane? Take three fifty-pound bags of feed, tie a rope around them, and then try to lift and carry all three any distance. Then lower that one hundred-fifty pound package gently onto a toilet seat in your bathroom. Hold the bags steady on the commode for five minutes. After that, move the bags into the shower. Wash down every square inch of the bags (assume they are waterproof) without letting them topple over. After you're finished, turn off the water while keeping the bags steady. Then dry them off and haul them gently onto the bed in the next room. Pull, push, tug, and lift the bags so they are positioned precisely and completely within a pre-traced outline on the sheets.

It isn't easy for a full-grown, strong man. Now consider that the two people who have been bench-pressing, squatting, and curling Duane for the last forty-six years are two women—his mother and his wife. It's no wonder they both have bad backs.

Taking care of an adult with SMA or MD is much harder than taking care of a child with the same disease.

First, the adult requires help much more frequently. Their muscles have deteriorated to the point that there is little they can do on their own. In other words, they need attention more often and for more reasons because they have little to no ability to move their limbs as they did when they were younger.

Because adult SMA'ers have no usable muscles to speak of, they cannot provide assisting or supplementary strength when they are being moved. If Kim tries to scoot Duane more upright in the bed, he can't wiggle, push his hand into the mattress, or do anything else to aid her.

Adults are bigger and heavier. That means they are a lot more difficult to move. Duane is one hundred and forty pounds of dead weight. He is no longer a fifty-pound kid who can be carried around by his father.

When Duane was ninety pounds and fourteen, he required help less often and with fewer tasks than he does today. When he did need help to move, his upper body was able to lend a little assisting strength to the helper. And, the caregiver had to manage ninety pounds of Duane instead of one hundred-forty. The amount of time and energy required to take care of Duane has increased every year for the past thirty-five years.

While working bedside with him on this project, one of the things that surprised me most was the forcefulness of the caregiving. I recall the expectations I had during my drive to his place for our first appointment. I pictured Kim gingerly raising him up, softly pushing his hips into position, easily swinging his legs around so he could get in his wheelchair. I envisioned a very tender process.

I was wrong.

There is nothing gentle, soft, or easy about moving Duane. When he needed to roll over, Logan got in the bed, curled up, put his feet against the wall, pressed a shoulder into his father's hip and grunted like a guy lifting weights at the gym who wants to be noticed as he rolled his dad's body over.

When Kim came home for lunch, she came into the bedroom, wrapped her arms under her husband's armpits, squeezed him in a bear hug, lifted, and raised him toward the headboard.

On top of the love, emotional support, caregiving and earning power she brings to the family, Kim is a physically strong woman. She must compensate for her husband's lack of strength. Few women have the muscle to do what she does. With her solid arms and powerful legs, she is not only emotionally equipped but also physically able to carry her family on her shoulders.

Turn Down Service

If I could have one minute of full movement, I would use it not to walk or run, but to embrace my wife.
--Duane

Human beings move while they sleep. Our minds sense the slightest discomforts, hot spots, pressure points, or tingles caused by reduced circulation. Without waking, our bodies respond to our brain's commands and roll around until we're comfortable. The process repeats itself all night long, until we awake in the morning, hopefully refreshed.

Duane doesn't just close his eyes and crash. There's a strict routine that has to be followed. As part of his turndown service, he has to be prepared for sleep.

Duane uses a special chair to move from his bed to the bathroom. After Kim gets him into that chair and pushes him into the bathroom, she raises the right armrest and places his elbow on it. She puts a toothbrush, bristles soaked in water and covered with toothpaste, in his elevated right hand. He slowly pokes the brush into his mouth and shakes his head back-and-forth and up-and-down to move his teeth along the bristles. The bobble-head doll imitation makes him a little dizzy, so he rests for a moment before turning his head and working the other side of his mouth.

Kim takes the toothbrush and replaces it with a disposable razor. She spreads shaving cream on his face. Duane presses the razor to a cheek and again moves his head in all kinds of directions. He's only able to mow down half the stubble by moving his skin under the razor. Kim finishes by shaving the patches he missed.

The ritual of shaving is one of those tasks in his transitory phase—something he used to do all on his own, but now can do only with other's help and great effort on his own part. Soon the act of shaving will join the ever-expanding list of things he used to do.

If neither his toenails nor fingernails require clipping, if his ears don't need cleaning, if he has no bedsores that need attention, it's time to use the restroom. When his bowel and bladder are empty, he's ready for his turn down service.

First, Kim lowers his side of their hospital-style bed from its thirty-degree, daytime incline to the horizontal position.

After she turns down the sheets and blankets, she either bearhugs Duane and lifts him from his chair to their bed or she uses the "Parham lift" to lift and lower him.

Standing beside the bed, she begins the process of getting her husband into his sleep-starting position—resting on his right side. She rolls Duane's hips over, then his shoulders so he's lying on his right side facing the outside of the bed. His head moves with his shoulders, but his legs don't move with his hips, so she rotates his always-bent-at-the-knees legs around so the full length of his left leg rests completely upon his right leg.

She hikes up his shoulders and head while wedging two pillows under his head. Then it's back to the legs. She raises his left leg and places a pillow between his knees. The leg pillow serves as padding to keep the bones in his knees from pressing against each other and creating hot spots. She lifts his head one more time and places a folded washcloth between the pillow and his temple to reduce the pressure which otherwise would build on his ear. The upper rim of his earlobe is one of the most sensitive parts of his body and over the years has proved to be prone to bedsores. Over the years, they've tried many different pads but have found nothing works as well as a folded washcloth.

Kim slides a towel between Duane's left elbow and his ribs. This will mitigate the hot spot created by his arm pressing into the side of his ribcage.

After the left arm is perfectly placed, she moves Duane's right arm, which is under his weight, placing his hand a few inches short of a thumb-sucking position. Then she puts the cordless phone at Duane's fingertips. Kim is a very heavy sleeper and the phone gives Duane functionality to call 911 or even to call Kim's phone on her side of the bed in the event he is unable to rouse her from sleep. He's able to move his right hand one inch to grip his cordless phone, which is placed in the same spot every night. He can't raise the phone to look at it or bring it to his head, but he can feel the keys and put it in speakerphone mode and make calls.

There is always the possibility Duane could wake in the middle of the night and have some kind of respiratory distress, laryngitis, or other ailment which prevents him from rousing Kim in a life-threatening emergency. It sounds ridiculous not to be able to wake up a person who is inches from you, but without the phone, Duane could wake in the middle of the night, smell smoke, and be completely helpless if his voice isn't strong enough to wake Kim.

Kim uses the remote to set the TV sleep timer on the TV for one hour. She lies down in the bed next to her husband and almost always falls asleep before he does. Duane takes a long time to doze off in his quasi-fetal position. He's not exactly comfortable, but as close to it as he can get.

He sleeps better during nights following days on which he gets out of the house. Getting out of bed, into his shell, moving into his chair, and then sitting erect for a few hours while buzzing around town has him physically exhausted at the end of the day. The intense physical demands of leaving the house and sitting erect is the primary reason that, in recent years, on some days he leaves his bed only to use the toilet. On those nights that follow days he has spent in bed, it's usually hard for him to fall asleep. If he has several days of inactivity, he's usually still awake when the TV clicks off, marking the end of his first hour of trying to fall asleep.

During the night, Duane's mind works just like ours. It tries to tell his body that it's time to roll over, to adjust positions. But his body can't respond. Like a defiant child, it does just the opposite of what it's told. It lays motionless.

You could surround Duane's entire, sleeping body with eggs and he wouldn't break a single one in his sleep.

● ● ●

His chest expands and contracts. His mouth may open or close and his nostrils will flare with each breath. His facial muscles might twitch. But other than that, Duane is a head on a manikin's body.

Eventually, his mind gets frustrated. Sick and tired of being ignored, it sounds a wakeup call to his body. His eyes open and he's in the exact same position he was when he fell asleep. The position that was comfortable enough two hours ago is now annoying him. His right hip is numb and tingling. His right shoulder has been pressed under his body weight without relief for too long and is heating up.

He knows if he tries to close his eyes and ignore the discomfort, the most he can hope for is twenty minutes of light sleep before his brain screams for adjustments. He wants to be moved. He wants a new position so he might sleep another hour. He has a choice to make. Does he wake his wife up now or suck it up for another half hour? He watches the clock move. He knows that if he can endure an extra thirty minutes it might translate to one less sleep interruption and a better night's rest for Kim. She gives him so much. This time, he'll close his eyes and try to milk his current position for just a little longer. This is his gift to her. One of the few things he can do for his wife—make a sacrifice to be uncomfortable to let her sleep.

A few minutes later, he wakes again. The right side of his ribs is pressing into the mattress and it burns. His right hip feels like it's resting in a bed of hot coals. The inside of his left knee is numbing. His earlobe has a dull ache. The collection of his pains has increased his discomfort to a point at which he knows he won't be able to doze off. He has reached his tolerance level. To push beyond would be torture. He looks at the clock. It's 2:10.

He has no choice; he has to wake Kim and get the adjustment. He starts calling her name with a soft voice.

"Kim?"

He knows it'll take a series of queries for her to respond. She sleeps like a rock. Each successive request gets a little louder, until he's almost shouting. Kim hears Duane's voice but interprets it as a dream. She still doesn't move. Eventually, whenever he does wake her, she may remember hearing her name and not responding.

Duane has learned that the sleeping Kim is often more responsive to words of things she fears.

Duane tries something else. "Bees, Bees! Kim, there's a bee on you!"

She still doesn't move.

He mocks her alarm clock. "Beep, beep, beep."

Duane can't wake her.

"Snake!" He yells almost as loud as he can. "Watch out for snakes!"

Logan hears his father from his bedroom. He dutifully comes into his parent's room, leans over his father's limp body and shakes his mother's shoulder. "Mom, dad needs tah move."

Her son's shake wakes Kim.

She whispers. "Thank you, Logan."

Logan pats his father on the shoulder and goes back to bed.

Kim knows what position her husband needs. They go through this every night—three hundred sixty-five nights a year. She practically reads his mind. She knows almost everything he needs.

There's only one thing she needs to ask. "You need to go pee?"

Duane responds softly. "No."

There's no need for any other verbal communication. A conversation would only make it more difficult for both of them to fall back into a slumber.

She starts by throwing the covers back and pulling the pillow out from between his legs. Sometimes she gets out of bed for better leverage, sometimes she tries to pull, tug, and roll him while she's in bed. She grips him under the armpits and lifts. She pushes his hips. She grabs him by the left shoulder and pulls hard. She does everything she did two hours when she had tucked him in to get him into a reciprocal position of the one he started in. When she is done, her husband will be lying on his left side, facing her.

The process takes about three or four minutes. When she's finished, she utters a question with a single word, "good?"

"Yes. Thank you, Kim."

His wife fades back to sleep quickly. Duane lies in bed and looks at his sleeping wife in the dark. He thanks God for her—for leading him to that rare woman whom he never thought he would find.

He wishes he could hug her. He longs to reach out and pull her body tight to his and stroke her arm softly with his fingers, to nuzzle his lips into the nape of her neck, to reciprocate the intimacy that moves between them almost exclusively in the direction of she to him. But his body will not move. Of all the functions it refuses to perform, its inability to obey this urge is one that is the hardest to accept. In almost every other regard he has learned to accept his disease and the limitations it has dealt him, but the inability to initiate a tender touch to his wife's body is perhaps the cruelest of all the disallowances of his disease.

Holding His Breath

Duane joined his friends in as many activities as he could. Swimming was his favorite sport. In fact, for several years after Duane had lost the strength to stand or walk, he could still do so in a swimming pool. Little muscle strength is required to walk in water or to float on top of it. Without heavy muscle mass, Duane could float better than anybody. Supported by the buoyancy of water, he could do almost everything everyone else did: Marco Polo, chicken fights, and play tag. He looked like everyone else while in the pool. If it were up to him he would have stayed in the pool all day. He especially liked to swim under water in his family's above-ground pool, trying to swim a whole lap without coming up for air.

One night while he and I were working on this manuscript, Ronald Bunch came over and joined me next to Duane's bed. Ronald had been Duane's best friend since sixth grade and was his "helper" at several summer MDA camps.

Duane started telling a story about an MDA camp he and Ronald had attended together the summer before eighth grade. Campers were broken up into teams and they competed in various competitions conducive to their disabilities, somewhat like the Special Olympics. One of the events was a contest in which each camper tried to hold their breath under water as long as they could.

I listened as Duane covered the smallest of details. "I had practiced holding my breath in the pool. Plus, I played the trumpet so that really helped my lungs. In fact, doctors told me I had the same lung capacity as healthy kids my age. I knew I had a good chance to win that contest."

A reflective smile spread across Duane's face as he bragged in a way I hadn't seen him do before. "Remember Ron, when I told you I was gonna win?"

Ronald throat-chuckled and nodded through his understated, tight-lipped grin.

Duane rambled on like a fisherman describing his biggest catch. "I sucked in as much air as I could and went under the same time as everyone else. I was holding the side of the concrete pool and with my eyes open underwater I saw everyone else come up one-by-one. How many kids were there, Ron, like fifteen?"

"Yeah, at least." Ron said.

Duane continued. "I was the last one still under when I heard voices talking from above."

Like some of Duane's other stories, I had decided by this point that there was nothing write-able about this. Although I saw how fond he was of reminiscing about it, I didn't see any way to capture the reader's interest in a trivial breathe-holding contest thirty-five years ago. Then, I noticed the knowing look on Ronald's face as he nodded a series of acknowledgements as Duane neared the end of his story. "I felt this hand try to raise me out of the water. I pushed it away."

❖ ❖ ❖

Duane looked at perhaps the only person in the world who shared his memory of the event. "You remember how they asked you if I was okay?"

Ronald's smiled grew a little bigger as he nodded again. "Oh yeah."

"I stayed under and raised my arm up out of the water and gave everyone a thumbs-up."

I could see the respect and pride in Ronald's eyes and he smiled while listening to his friend's account of a rare sports triumph. It was the kind of look one might see on a father who's watching his son round the bases after hitting a home run.

"How long did I stay under, Ron? Like a minute or something?"

"A minute-twenty," Ronald recalled. Clearly the event was as memorable to Ronald as it was to Duane. If Duane was this animated about a contest he won so long ago, I could only imagine how excited he must have been when it happened.

Ron's expression made me understand that from Duane's point of view, winning that breath-holding competition was no different to him than my memories of my great sports moments.

Most of us have those kind of memories or glory days, even if we weren't good athletes: A girl who made one basket in seventh grade all season long then never played again, a boy who almost always struck out but on one occasion closed his eyes and hit a solid line drive that won the game.

You don't have to be a great athlete to have a great athletic moment. And to Duane, someone who never played organized sports, those eighty seconds underwater were his greatest athletic moment. He won a flag for his team and that breath-holding contest would forever be the closest he'd ever come to experiencing the thrill of athletic victory. It seemed to me that Duane sharing that singular, champion moment with his best friend meant as much to Ronald as it did to Duane.

Duane Is Funny

Somehow, Duane has figured out how to live a happy and fulfilling life. Nothing seems to please him more than someone listening to him talk. He'll talk to anyone who listens. In fact, he won't shut up. If you ever engage Duane in a discussion, be advised, he lacks an exit strategy to his conversations.

While working on this project, I'd often debate whether to call or email him to get the answer to a single question. *Well...he is probably just sitting in bed. It'd probably give him a warm, fuzzy feeling to know that I'm working on the book. But, I'm not going to let him suck me in for another half hour. I'll get my answer, and then get back to writing.* Rarely did that strategy work.

I made a phone call to ask him a simple question. "Duane, which kids carried you piggyback besides Les?"

Here is how he answered that question: "Hey…you know, I saw Les at Chilis Monday night. Guess who he said came into Lowes together to buy a dishwasher?"

An hour later, after getting caught up on how Les' sister is doing in Germany and hearing a rundown on every friend he had added to Facebook in the last two days, I'd ask him the same question again.

“Duane, I gotta write. Let me go, dude, or we’ll never finish your book.”

Have you ever heard someone claim blind people become so reliant on their ears that they tend to develop an acute sense of hearing? Duane talks so much because he has been deprived of so much else. His arms and legs don’t work, so his mouth has to make up for it.

He can be pretty funny. The first time I came in his room I asked him how he was doing.

“I’m having a bad day. See that remote an inch from my right hand? It slid out of my reach this morning and I’ve been stuck watching the Home Shopping Network for the last four hours.”

He has collected some pretty good one-liners. Call him and ask him what he’s doing.

“Oh I was just out jogging.”

Ask him about his schedule.

“Let me see here…uhm…Monday, I’ll be in bed…and ahh…Tuesday…looks like bed all day. And Wednesday, I’ll be in bed all day until Logan’s baseball game at five.

When Logan forgets to do a chore he makes his point with humor.

“Logan, don’t make me get up and spank you.”

When he and Kim get into a minor argument, he might bring it to a quick end by threatening her. “Kim, don’t make me walk out on you.”

Duane has every right to be withdrawn and miserable. But he isn’t. Duane is funny.

* * *

The Cure

If one watches documentaries, reads blogs and on-online discussions or talks to SMA families they will hear a common thread from parents. The hardest thing for them to accept about their child's disease is their powerlessness. No amount of physical therapy, money, commitment, effort, willpower, medicine, or parental love can alter the inescapable future of their children. They all want to fight, but the fight is fixed, the judges have been paid off. They are utterly helpless. All they can do is hope for a cure. Just like the previous generations of SMA parents, as long as their son or daughter is alive, their hope is eternal.

Every mother and father wishes they could trade places with their SMA child. They take their children to doctors, physical therapists, camps and workshops, buy wheelchairs and vans and convert their homes to accommodate their children's needs, all the while hoping and praying for a cure. Many parents leave their old lives behind, giving up virtually all hobbies and interests they once had to take care of their children 24/7. Even while doing all of that, they often blame themselves for the single defective gene they passed on. Just like the previous generations of SMA parents, their guilt and anguish is eternal.

Today's SMA families are on the Internet, combing through scientific journals trying to make sense of the thirteen-letter words they read describing the results of clinical trials of experimental therapies on mice. They learn that SMA mice in labs all over the world are jumping out of their wheelchairs and running to wedges of cheese. Meanwhile they can only sit and wait for the slow and often bureaucratic and political machinery of alphabet soup organizations like the NIH and FDA to approve the start of meaningful human trials.

Those SMA parents all have the same question: When the cure comes, will it be too late for my child? Is there any chance for my son or daughter to be cured? Meanwhile, they love their children with all their might because for now, that's all they can offer them. Just like the previous generations of SMA parents, their love is eternal.

There is no cure for SMA, but progress toward one is very promising. You'll find advocates who speak those words about almost every disease. For SMA, the hope is not hollow lip service. It is based upon facts and results more than emotions. There's a consensus among experts that researchers are on the verge of a breakthrough treatment. The National Institute for Health, NIH, has selected SMA for a pilot project in translational research based in large part because SMA offers a high probability for the development of a treatment or cure. Even a well-informed skeptic would agree a cure is imminent. More money is needed, not a lot of money, just a few hundred million dollars or so might be enough to put an end to this terrible disease.

It will soon be thirty-five years since Duane last walked. Given his age and his stage of the illness, he knows it's unlikely that a cure or any treatment for the disease will benefit him personally. "I used to be consumed with the prospects of a cure. I used to dream of the day I would get up and walk. It's easy for those kinds of dreams to become an obsession. I think most MDA and SMA people spend a lot of time wishing they were healthy and visualizing a life they don't have. I used to live that kind of alternate life in my fantasies to the point that I decided it was diminishing the quality of the life I did have. Having hope for a cure is healthy, but unless it's balanced with acceptance, it's easy to get demoralized and curl up and withdraw. If you let yourself succumb to resentment or pity, you will be miserable. I decided long ago that I wasn't going to let that happen to me."

If

Over forty years ago doctors told the parents of a cute, little, blonde curly-haired, four-year-old boy that their son would probably not live past his teens. A few years later, that boy decided he wanted to prove those doctors wrong. He set a goal to graduate high school. He blew through that objective and spent the next three decades setting and achieving new goals.

He found a career, learned to drive, bought a house, helped save lives, got married, had a son, provided for his family, and became a good father. To a healthy man, his dreams may seem simple but to a man with no muscles, those same ambitions once seemed unreasonable, even unattainable.

Today, as he puts a bow on yet another goal—to write a book and share his story—he looks toward his next one: to see his son graduate high school.

If he were born today, maybe the answer to his parent's question, "Will the cure come too late for my child?" Would be "no."

Perhaps, if Duane Hale were born with SMA-3 today, forty-six years from now there would be nothing remarkable to write about him. Maybe he would take a few shots every so often but otherwise be in the midst of an average, typical life.

If Duane Hale were born today, he might not have to fight so hard to achieve *normal*. Without that fight, a today-born-Duane might turn out to be an ordinary man instead of the one he became.

About the Authors

Rich Ochoa – Lindale High Class of '82

To ensure you're notified when his next book is published, and to learn more about Rich Ochoa, he invites you to friend request him on *Facebook.*

He'd also like it if you "liked" the books, *One Way Ticket to Anywhere* and *Life Rolls On The Book* on *Facebook.* Hardcore fans may even follow him on *Twitter.* For sample chapters of his ongoing projects, visit **onewaytickettoanywhere.com.**

Duane Hale - Lindale High Class of '83

I am proud to have grown up in Lindale, Texas. Although many of my friends are not mentioned by name in this book, I cherish each one.

I grew up as a normal child but I knew that I was different. Life has been a challenge but I wouldn't change anything. The struggles I went through as a child only made me stronger.

Thank you Rich, for helping tell my story. Working on the project with you has been therapeutic, enriching, and one of the most enjoyable times of my life.

To anyone who reads this book, feel free to leave feedback on amazon.com. Five star reviews help the book climb the charts (smiling as I write). Also feel free to contact me through my Facebook page or email me at iiceman@yahoo.com. Please "like" the Facebook page,

Families of Spinal Muscular Atrophy. And support all efforts to find a cure for this disease.

Also by Rich Ochoa

One Way Ticket to Anywhere

RICH'S mother kicks him out of the house in a drunken fury when he refuses to eat kidney beans. The sixteen year old is put on a bus and rides cross-country to meet his father, whom he had been conditioned to fear as the monster who abducted him as an infant. Two months later, his stepmother offers him a one-way bus ticket to anywhere he wants to go.

After perusing a road atlas for a place to finish high school, the protagonist devises a plan. He'll "Go Greyhound" from Idaho to his former hometown, Lindale, Texas. He'll build a fort in the woods behind the high school where he'll sleep until he can land a job, cash some paychecks and find a room to rent.

As he steps onto the bus and into adulthood, he counts his belongings as twenty dollars cash, fifty dollars of food stamps and a garbage bag full of clothes.

Available on Amazon and Barnes & Noble

CPSIA information can be obtained
at www.ICGtesting.com
Printed in the USA
LVOW12s1007270318
571311LV00001B/10/P